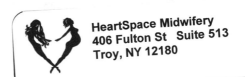

Birthrites

Rituals and celebrations for
the child-bearing years

About the Author

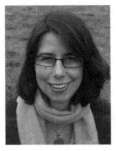 Jackie Singer studied English at Oxford University, and then trained as a Drama and Movement Therapist at the Central School of Speech and Drama in London. Over the next fifteen years she led creative and therapeutic projects with a wide variety of community groups in Oxfordshire, and honed her skills as a musician and storyteller.

Jackie has always found ritual important for marking the significant changes in her own life, and helpful for moving through difficult times. In 2001 she began offering her services as a celebrant to facilitate other people to experience the benefits of non-denominational ceremony. Improvisation as a route to inspiration is a common thread in all her work.

Jackie now lives in Oxford with her husband and two young children, and divides her time between writing, making ceremonies, playing music, telling stories, and changing nappies.

Birthrites

Rituals and celebrations for the child-bearing years

Jackie Singer

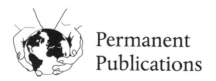

Permanent
Publications

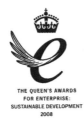

THE QUEEN'S AWARDS
FOR ENTERPRISE:
SUSTAINABLE DEVELOPMENT
2008

Published by

Permanent Publications
Hyden House Ltd
The Sustainability Centre
East Meon
Hampshire GU32 1HR
United Kingdom
Tel: 01730 823 311
Fax: 01730 823 322
Overseas: (international code +44 - 1730)
Email: enquiries@permaculture.co.uk
Web: www.permaculture.co.uk

This publication is kindly supported by

The Green Parent Magazine, PO Box 104, East Hoathley, Lewes BN7 9AX
Tel: 01825 872 858 Email: info@thegreenparent.co.uk Web: info@the greenparent.co.uk

First edition © 2009 Jackie Singer

The right of Jackie Singer to be identified as the author of this work has been asserted by her in accordance with the Copyrights, Designs and Patents Act 1998

Drawings by Imogen Oxley

Designed by Two Plus George Limited, www.TwoPlusGeorge.co.uk

Printed in the UK by Cambrian Printers, Aberystwyth

Paper from FSC certified mixed sources

FSC
Mixed Sources
Product group from well-managed
forests and other controlled sources
Cert no. TF-COC-2200
www.fsc.org
© 1996 Forest Stewardship Council

The Forest Stewardship Council (FSC) is a non-profit international organisation established to promote the responsible management of the world's forests. Products carrying the FSC label are independently certified to assure consumers that they come from forests that are managed to meet the social, economic and ecological needs of present and future generations.

British Library Cataloguing-in-Publication Data

A catalogue record for this book is available from the British Library

ISBN 978 1 85623 049 0

Dedication

For Sheila and Geoffrey, the ones who stand behind me

And Heather and Penny, the ones I shall stand behind

Contents

Thanks

My thanks go firstly to all the contributors, whose stories give life to this book. To the friends who read drafts and offered feedback at various stages, especially Matilda Leyser, Adèle Moss and Kate Mohideen. Special thanks to Janet Stansfeld and Jo Hamilton for their long-standing encouragement. To Wren and Richard Hughes and Jonquil Bennet, who offered peaceful places to write. To my parents-in-law Jacquie and Mike Pritchard and Lesley Papper, who helped take care of the children and Efda Koci who kept the house in order. To Maddy and Tim Harland, my editors, for being excellent collaborators. To Paula Jacobs, whose gentle wisdom has made its way into much of this book. To my novelist sister Nicky for all that she has shared. Finally to my husband Phil, for embarking on the journey of making a family with me.

Foreword by Glennie Kindred

We are living in extraordinary times of change, both in our relationship with the Earth and in our relationships with each other. We are seeking ways to change ourselves, to adapt and move from our old outworn belief systems, to create new ways forward that are true reflections of our present day understanding. We are changing the way we think. We no longer see ourselves as separate from our experiences, each other or the Earth but as part of a beautiful interconnected web of life. We are becoming aware that everything we do affects the complex balance of our minds, emotions and our physical health as well as that of the natural world around us. We can look back on our past and see the patterns and beliefs that have brought us to this point. We may be filled with despair and grief for all that has been damaged and lost but once we fully acknowledge this, we are able to find ways to move on and begin to take the steps towards healing the past and creating new ways to live in the present.

Ceremony and ritual fulfil a natural need and longing to make connection to the deeper levels of ourselves and the inter-dimensional awareness and spirituality that is an inherent part of us all. Through them we are more able to understand the complex web of our lives and the world we live in. They help us to slow down, to listen to our hearts, to acknowledge our feelings, our thoughts, and intuitive wisdom.

This helps us to become stronger, clearer in our direction and healthier, ready to move on to the next stage of our lives.

Jackie Singer is part of a growing movement of pioneers who are finding new ways of marking the life changing moments we all have. In this book she explores and shares her experiences, and the experiences of many others, to create open and inclusive ceremonies and rituals to honour the experience of birth. She comprehensively looks at ways to mark its many stages, before and after the birth and also includes ways to mark the many complex related aspects of unfulfilled dreams and death.

With a very accessible style of writing, Jackie draws on the past, on different cultural traditions and faiths and also acknowledges an open-hearted loving spirituality that has no name or label. She reveals the common components of any ceremony and ritual so we are able to devise our own or work with a celebrant. She encourages us to be courageous, to be creative, inventive and experimental. She inspires us to find ways to make these ceremonies inclusive and heartfelt. She inspires us to trust our instincts and the great gift of trusting our friends and our community to support us, to celebrate or to grieve with us and to bear witness. At this grass roots level we take our power firmly in our own hands to create lasting and memorable moments and experiences that bring connection, joy, inner peace and healing into our lives and into the lives of our families and the friends we share them with.

Glennie Kindred
Author, artist and celebrant
September 2009

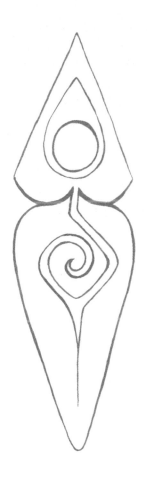

Introduction

Very quietly, behind closed doors, men and women everywhere are making life and death decisions. We pop a pill, we put on a condom, or we throw caution to the wind. Behind other doors, people are dissolving into the bliss of gazing at their newborn babies. Behind still other doors, there are those who are silently grieving for the children that died before they were born, for abortions they never came to terms with, for fertility treatment that didn't work out. For the most part, we feel embarrassed about feeling so much, and are quick to get back to work. Yet these changes are profound and the feelings are overwhelming. This is humanity at its most glorious and vulnerable. Surely these things are worthy of a little more of our attention?

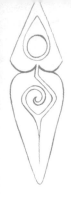

One way to connect with the deeper currents of what is happening here physically, emotionally, mentally and spiritually is through ritual. Whether we have a need to express joy and celebration or to grieve our losses, rituals give us time to pause, gather our community around us, and dive below the surface of day-to-day life to engage with the deeper mysteries of birth, death and transformation. Far from being only the province of the religious traditions, ritual is a way of thinking and working that is accessible to everyone. In our times, many ordinary people are finding ways to answer their own needs by forging rituals. *Birthrites* tells their stories, and provides practical encouragement to anyone wishing to use ritual as a way to navigate the vast and unpredictable waters of their fertility.

My own fascination with ritual owes much to my family. I was the youngest of five, and my mother had a great sense of occasion; from her I learnt the importance of marking birthdays and festivals. Then again, my mother's determination that life should be celebrated was probably part of the way she dealt with bringing up a large family alone after the sudden death of her husband when I was a nine-month-old baby. The rituals of grief were less well understood in our household. When she herself died of cancer, I was a seventeen-year-old with an urgent need to question life deeply, and a turbulent swell of emotions to express. For me, the big questions – Where do we come from? What is life for? Where do we go when we die? – were not idle philosophy but my most pressing concerns. With this background, it is probably not surprising that I gravitated towards working with people in a form that gives a context big enough to contain all of our individual human joys and sorrows. From using ritual to help in my own life, and researching these practices,

I began to work as a celebrant, supporting others in the creation of meaningful ceremonies for themselves.

The places in which I have learnt about ritual and working with spirit, have been various. As a child, I was a devout Christian, happy to accept 'my father in heaven', and equipped with a cheerful song or rousing hymn for every occasion. I was confirmed in the Church of England, despite presenting my school chaplain with awkward questions. In student years, I oscillated uncomfortably between evangelical episodes and profound doubting. Finally throwing religion off, I was rationally an atheist, but then fell in love, experimented with psychedelics, kept company with T. S. Eliot, discovered Rumi, and almost went mad with Virginia Woolf. Much flailing ensued, during which I nearly failed to complete my English degree. A little later, studying C. G. Jung as part of my drama and movement therapy training gave me a bigger picture. Then I found a local Quaker group, began celebrating the seasonal festivals with Pagans, and found myself singing and dancing with a community of people who celebrated the spirit of the earth. I learnt about Native American ceremony as adapted by Celtic iconoclasts in the Welsh hills. When my sister had a crisis I enquired about a retreat centre on her behalf, which, years later, ended up becoming my own spiritual home – halfway up a Herefordshire mountain with a Sufi meditation teacher. Here I found an introduction to the divine feminine; a kind of prayer that included walking, moving and singing, and a faith that seemed big enough to encompass everything else. Throughout all this seeking, making music and improvisation has often been my most direct line to inspiration. You may surmise from this that my concepts of god, goddess, prayer, worship, spirit and ritual are

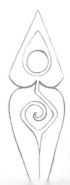

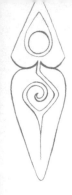

somewhat broad. For the time being at any rate, I have given up trying to analyse and define things, and am growingly content to pray, trust, and acknowledge the depth of my unknowing. As Louis MacNeice memorably put it: "World is crazier and more of it than we think."[1]

I began writing this book from the perspective of someone who had not yet crossed the threshold into motherhood, although for many years I had longed to. Perhaps because motherhood did not come quickly or easily for me, I spent longer than most considering what it means, thinking about how I might confront infertility, and if I would choose to adopt a child. Just as I was putting the finishing touches to the first draft, I discovered I was pregnant. Two years later, with an ebullient toddler and a six-month-old baby in the house, I returned to integrate my new experiences into the manuscript.

* * *

The book begins with a short exploration of what ritual is, followed by two chapters which set out some practical pointers for people thinking about organising an event. The main body of the book is organised by theme, so that you can turn directly to the chapter of most interest to you at any moment.

Early chapters look at preparations for couples who are thinking of having a child, and rituals to do during pregnancy and birth. There are descriptions of ceremonies where people have come together specifically to celebrate a pregnancy and help a woman prepare for birth. There are contributions by men who have chosen to mark their transition into fatherhood in some particular way. Many of these are not public ceremonies; rather they are small but significant thoughts, words, or actions, which people have performed privately and spontaneously. I include them because they are all part of an approach that treats the experience of birth as a rite of passage.

A central chapter looks at welcoming and naming babies. The arrival of a child is a natural cause for celebration within the community; many parents, who may or may not feel part of a religious tradition, yearn to mark the birth and naming of their child in some way, whether it's by planting a tree or sailing origami boats down the river.

An investigation into fertility and birth would not be complete without the painful journeys that many individuals or couples face, when conception doesn't come easily, or a pregnancy doesn't come to full term. Our society offers some startling medical interventions, which can result in great successes, but has less to offer people dealing with the emotional burden of miscarriage, stillbirth or infertility. These things can even be seen as medical failures. Ritual can be particularly helpful at such moments as a way of giving space to engage with difficult feelings and to reach beyond ourselves for support.

Some families are created by adoption, with the experience of pregnancy and labour replaced by an arduous passage through assessments and legal procedures. The chapter on adoption de-scribes ceremonies for adoptive parents wishing to create a warm and memorable welcome for their adopted child. Remembering the other two points of the adoption triangle, rituals of mourning are considered for the natural parents who have given up a child for adoption, and suggestions are made for the adopted child struggling to make sense of their own identity.

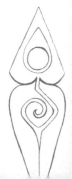

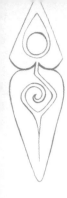

Whatever our views about it, termination of a pregnancy is a fact in our society. Rituals are offered here to help those who choose this path with dignity and awareness. There are also those who, for different reasons, choose not to have children. Their stories, and the ways they have supported themselves in their decisions, form the last part of the picture of this stage of life.

At the end of the book you will find an extensive collection of resources. I would have liked to include more poems in this book, but sadly copyright law makes this prohibitively expensive. Instead I have listed a number of relevant poems and songs arranged by chapter, and given details of how to find them. I also suggest some excellent anthologies and sourcebooks for poems, prayers and readings. There is also a list of recommended books for further reading, and details of organisations which offer support and information on a range of issues. Finally, I have included a list of celebrants who can be contacted to help devise or hold an event. As yet, there is no national directory of freelance celebrants, so this is a partial list of people whose work is known to me personally and whom I feel glad to recommend.

* * *

The richness of this book derives from the real-life stories of all kinds of people, who have gone about developing rituals in their own individual ways. These include people from particular faiths who have broken new ground by inventing a ritual they felt was not provided by their tradition, as well as individuals who have no church and were reaching for a new language of word or symbol to express their meaning. The rituals themselves range in size, from community events, such as baby naming celebrations, through to private practices or silent meditations. Some express a profoundly spiritual perspective on life; others represent exemplary ways to deal with the inner emotional work of being human.

Particularly in the latter half of the book, in dealing with those stages of life that are not covered by mainstream ritual, I have offered structures and words for rituals of my own devising. I have tried to use open language when writing these in the hope of reaching people of many faiths or none. All of these frameworks are intended to be inspirational, not prescriptive. Occasionally I have suggested a prayer addressed to either a non-gendered or a feminine expression of divinity, such as 'Spirit of Life' or 'Compassionate Mother'. These are names that I have found helpful, but clearly, if you are used to addressing a particular deity, it will be natural for you to use their name instead. If not, you could experiment until you find a name that means something to you. If you are a woman and you are not used to addressing God as a female, I urge you to try it, and visualise her smiling, with open arms to hold you. Above all, I encourage you to improvise, as I have done, and find what works for you. At worst, you might feel a little silly. At best, you will tap a deep vein of human wisdom, which will nourish you and others.

In researching this book, I have had the pleasure of talking to dozens of people who have entrusted me with their intimate stories. Some were known to me personally, others were friends of friends, and some answered an advertisement to help with my research. Each one has taught me something, and I am indebted to them all for their courage and inspiration. To preserve confidentiality, names of individuals have been changed. I also pay tribute to all the celebrants

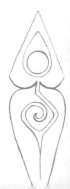

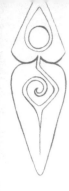

and professionals who have generously shared their thoughts and experiences. These people are named, and their contact details can be found in the Resources section.

Whilst I have aimed to cover many of the life events that can occur during the child-bearing years, I am aware that this is not a comprehensive account, and there will undoubtedly be gaps and biases. There is certainly scope for more exploration of how people are dealing with the fast-moving science of infertility treatments. There are many more stories from women than men, a disproportionate reference to people in couples rather than single parents, and very little from the point of view of same sex couples.

This is not from a desire to exclude anybody; I hope I have given enough examples and ideas that people in all kinds of family set-ups will be able to ignore what is not relevant, and find inspiration and encouragement to design rituals that work for them. Creating new ceremony is a work in progress to which individuals are contributing all the time. If you have a story to tell that would improve the balance for a second edition I would be pleased to hear from you.

Lastly, this book is intended to be the first of four books covering rituals for the four stages of life: Birth, Youth (including coming of age), Adulthood (including marriage, and divorce) and Elders (including menopause, retirement and funerals). If you have an experience you would like to share in any of these areas, please feel free to get in touch.

js@jackiesinger.co.uk

Chapter 1

Making Ritual

"Caminante, no hay camino, se hace camino al andar"
(Traveler, there is no path. One makes the path by walking.)
Antonio Machado[2]

Making ritual is a distinctly human behaviour. Like all other animals, humans are born, grow into adulthood, mate, produce young and die, but unlike other animals, we feel the need to gather together and mark these moments with ritual. As conscious beings, it seems we need time to process and integrate the seminal changes that happen to us. Making ritual diverts our attention from the everyday tasks of survival, and for a brief time allows us to notice and comment on where we are. Faced with the awesome experience of finding ourselves conscious in an unpredictable universe, making ritual is a noble attempt to confer rhythm and coherence on our lives.

For some, a ritual is a useful framework within which to contain strong emotions; for others it is a conversation with the gods. In either case, ritual works through a poetry of doing. It is a multi-sensory experience; often with music, dancing, dressing up, rich scents, special foods and symbols, which enter deeply into the body's memory. It makes bridges between the inner world of dreams, feelings, and potential, and the outer world of manifest reality. We use ritual as a language to tell our bodies and souls something that our minds already know, and we also use ritual to try to understand something that our bodies and souls are telling us.

Ritual is a powerful tool, which has been used for destructive ends as well as for good. When used to mark rites of passage, the significant beginnings and endings in our lives, it lends a majesty to our unfolding, letting each individual know they are valued within their community and part of the human family. At times of grief, ritual offers a container that is deep and strong enough to hold intense emotion.

Yet for many reasons, rituals in our modern society are greatly impoverished. Modern man has believed himself so rational that he can dismiss ritual as mumbo jumbo. We are so obsessed with 'getting on' we find it hard to stop our economic activities and pay attention to these profound inner changes. Instead of affirming the lives of each humble individual, we prefer to lavish attention on a select few celebrities, whose success is at the expense of everyone else. We often lack a local community, which makes it harder to gather together. And while the churches, mosques and synagogues cater for some of the population, many of us lack a shared belief-system that would make plain what should be done. Even within religious traditions, society is moving so fast that the rituals of the past may not be appropriate for the demands of the day.

In this context some significant rites of passage have disappeared altogether, and others have become reduced to a dry civil transaction, which tells you your place in society, but cannot make the heart sing. There are vestiges of ritual in house-warming parties and baby showers, and in greetings cards for birthdays and anniversaries, but these are generally a far cry from the soul food that is needed if we are to thrive rather than merely survive.

However, the urge to create ritual seems to be resilient in the face of all these changes. From time to time we hear a story that chimes a bell as if from far back in the memory. A mother spontaneously buys her son a necklace when his voice breaks. A man takes off on a pilgrimage to mark his fiftieth birthday. A woman tenderly wraps a carving in a length of seaweed and throws it into the sea to say goodbye to her miscarried child. Meanwhile, humanists are reworking ceremonies without God and there is a surge of interest in earth-based shamanic and indigenous practises. More and more people now have the courage and confidence to devise their own rituals in their own words.

Of course there is a paradox inherent in the whole concept of new ceremony, because part of the power of ceremony is that it has the weight of tradition behind it. In times of continuity, ritual would be something handed down by the elders. Perhaps this is an ideal, but we do not live in times of continuity. Rather than abandoning the whole idea of ritual as irrelevant, we need to respond to the challenges of our fast-changing age by renewing ritual practise in a way that honours the past but makes sense to us now.

Psychologically and emotionally, human beings still need ritual. Part of our brains may be modern and rational, but part is still childlike, thinks in pictures and is comforted by actions rather than words. We still need to step outside our individual busyness and place ourselves in a bigger context, to be in touch with the community of the ancestors, and the ones to come. And just as much as our ancestors once did, we still need inspiration to turn the base metal of our lives into something noble. As to how, there is not one answer, but a multitude of creative responses. The pouring out of inspiration, spirit, love, and guidance is a never-drying fountain, to which we can come to take a draught. Making ritual is like forging a cup. The cup may be ornate or plain, polished or rough, but if we take our cup to the fountain, the spirit will still fill it.

Chapter 2

Elements of Ceremony

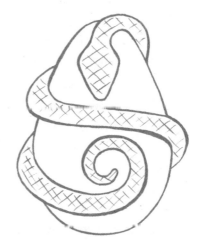

However public or private our ritual, there are certain things it is helpful to bear in mind when considering how to make a ceremony that functions well. This chapter takes a look at some of the elements that are common to ceremonies of all kinds.

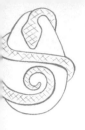

Shape

Like a good story, a satisfying ritual has a beginning, a middle and an end. There is a kind of dramatic tension that builds during the event, is relieved at the climax of the ritual, and is followed by celebration.

At the beginning, we make a transition from our normal life to this special occasion. We may choose particular clothes to wear and enter a ceremonial space. As we enter, silence or music may greet our ears, and incense may help to awaken us to a new state. We will be welcomed and reminded of the purpose of the ritual. This is also the time when spiritual helpers may be invoked to be present at the ritual; Druids call in the Four Directions, Anglicans say prayers to Almighty God and Quakers sit in silence waiting upon guidance from within.

There may be all kinds of songs and readings leading up to the moment in the ritual where the deed that everyone came there to witness is performed: for instance, the baby's head is anointed, vows are pronounced, a threshold is irrevocably passed over.

From that moment, the mood relaxes; there may be further music, words or blessings leading up to the closure of the ceremony. Guests are thanked and usually invited to join in feasting and celebration. If spirits were evoked, they too are thanked and released. The ending is marked in some way – from a jubilant fanfare to a simple handshake.

It seems obvious to state this order of events, but I have witnessed an occasion where the party happened first, and a ceremony was tacked onto the end almost as an afterthought. Both the party and the ceremony suffered as a result.

Sacred Time

A kind of magic happens when a number of people put a date in their diaries: a piece of the fabric of time starts to be held open for a purpose, and a container is formed. The original meaning of the word 'sacred' is 'set aside', so in this most basic sense, the time set aside from the daily round of economic activities can be said to be sacred. But there is also a deeper meaning to this. A powerful ritual brings us into the realm of the eternal, where time becomes elastic and an hour can morph into a landscape with a wide-open horizon. If we are moving in this realm, doing work that connects us with both our ancestors and the ones to come, we truly enter a time outside, or possibly inside, time. In order to dive into this 'dreamtime', we need to protect ourselves from intrusions and interruptions. Something as simple as switching off the TV, radio, computer and telephone for a while can make a profound difference.

A number of the things I suggest in this book may take a bit of time to do. Dreaming up a ceremony, making decorations rather than buying balloons, walking to a venue rather than driving door to door – all of these things require us to slow down, and experience what we are doing. This is a major challenge in our speed-addicted society. Yet any time we spend celebrating our passage through life and supporting our friends to do the same is richly repaid. It is the satisfaction of a homemade pie rather than a takeaway pizza, a meal that will go on nourishing the spirit for as long as the memories last. Having said that, a swiftly performed deed with a clear intention can also be powerful, and sometimes a visualisation alone is enough. Especially given the demands of life with small children, we need to bear in mind the art of the possible, rather than aiming for perfection.

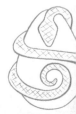

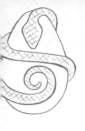

A further aspect of sacred time is the rhythm we give to our lives when we mark rites of passage. When we make a ceremony, we shoot an arrow of intention into the future, and start walking towards it. The first anniversary of a ceremony is a significant time when the results of the work we have done come to fruition, often in ways we could never have predicted. Further anniversaries may also continue to resonate with the energy of the work we have done.

Sacred Space

Choosing a space for a ceremony often brings us into contact in the first instance with caretakers, booking clerks or landowners. These people are the guardians of a place, and it is important that they understand what we want to do and are happy for us to be there. If this primary relationship is not harmonious, it will be hard to feel welcome, however lovely the environment.

Some places are already full of calm energy that helps to centre us the moment we arrive. In a building, this presence comes about not by accident but by layer upon layer of prayer and stillness. Some places in nature have an inherent genius locus. We are lucky when we have access to such places. I have been in chapels, caves, wooded glades and Quaker Meeting Houses where the presence of the place was so palpable, it called me instantly to reverence. In these places, the space prepares us more than the other way around.

More often than not, we need to work to prepare a space for welcoming people and containing our ritual. A community hall may well have been used for a playgroup, a boxing class, and a public meeting in the last week and echoes of those activities will still be bouncing around the walls. To make it sacred to our purpose, we need to clean and clear not just the physical clutter, but also the energetic detritus. This is like washing up a cooking pot before we start to add our ingredients.

One way to do this is by burning dried herbs; a practice used by indigenous groups the world over. I sometimes use a sage bundle. I like the fact that a bundle usually lasts a while, so lighting it again reminds me of the other times I've done ritual work. Native Americans use white sage, which is associated with removing negative energy, cedar for purification, and sweet-grass for positive energy. Of herbs that grow in this country, Lavender has a calming and uplifting effect, green or purple Sage is good for cleansing and Rosemary is useful for protection and mental clarity. You can buy smudge sticks from all kinds of suppliers or make your own from garden herbs.[3]

To make a herb bundle you will need fresh herbs, strong thread and a piece of thick fabric for rolling the herbs. Cut bunches of fresh lavender and rosemary in lengths of around 6 inches, and tie the ends together with strong thread. Wrap the thread around the bundle tightly, going all the way to the tips of the branches and then back again, criss-crossing over the first threads. Tie the threads off tightly at the bottom. Place the bundle inside the fabric, and roll forwards and backwards a few times. Finally hang it in a dry, shady place to dry.

When you are ready to cleanse the space, light your smudge stick or herb bundle until it flares and then blow it out so that the herbs are just smouldering. Hold in your mind your intention to cleanse the space and, if you like, ask the herbs for their help. If you would like to use herbs in a place where smoke is not a good idea (some public halls have sensitive fire alarm systems) you could add a

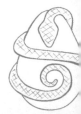

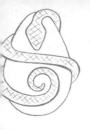

few drops of essential oils to a bottle of water in a spray-mist bottle and use this instead.

Having done this, a hall is easily transformed by softening the lighting, bringing in flowers or greenery, and hanging banners. Taking down these decorations and restoring the room to its original purpose is a part of the closing of the ritual, and should also be done with care and respect for the place.

If you are working at home, you could simply clear a space in a room, cover the computer, TV and paperwork with a cloth, put up a 'Please don't disturb' sign and unplug the 'phone. Some people like to create a circle around themselves, for example with cloths, stones or anything easily to hand. Herbs or essential oils can then be used as above.

Making an Altar

At its most basic, an altar is any structure holding items that the person who made it deems sacred. A home may have a permanent altar, such as a shelf or table, on which are placed significant and beautiful objects, photographs, pictures, religious icons or the text of prayers. In a sense, your mantelpiece may inadvertently have become an altar, if you use it to display objects that inspire you and photographs of loved ones. Once you have set up an altar, you can bring in fresh flowers or greenery to renew the altar and make it relevant to the day and season. Lighting a candle, or burning incense, animates the altar for a period of time during meditation or ritual work. Candlelight and incense appeal strongly to the senses, and make an environment conducive to prayer and reflection. If used regularly for this purpose they begin to act as triggers for a quieter state of mind.

A temporary altar may also be made as a focal point for a meditation or ceremony. In this case the base and objects will be relevant to the purpose of the event. There are no limits to creativity in choosing how to make an altar or what to put on it. I have made altars outdoors on tree stumps, rocks and the earth. Indoors, I like to choose a cloth as the base, with a colour that suits the purpose of the ritual. It doesn't have to be a special piece of fabric; a scarf, tablecloth, or item of clothing can be pressed into service. On top I have arranged, at different times, stones, leaves, flowers, fruit, a bowl of water, rice and beans, and even a lump of snow. But that list reveals my tendency to appreciate Spirit through the beauty of Nature. You could equally use tinsel and fairy lights.

If you are making an altar for a group activity, everyone can light a small candle to affirm their participation, or bring a personal item (a ring or a pendant, for example) to put on the altar. In shamanic practice, it is said that these things pick up the vibrational energy of the ritual and hold it for time to come.

Making an altar can be very satisfying. For one thing, it is an intensely creative activity, and it requires no particular skill to make something beautiful. But it is more than this. The Sufis have a song: "This is my body; this is the temple of light. This is my heart; this is the altar of love". In essence, an altar is a symbol of the heart, on which we make our offerings to the Beloved. If you prefer, you can simply visualise making a journey to the heart, dusting off the cobwebs, arranging fresh flowers and tending the flame of the eternal candle within.

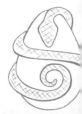

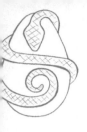

Purification

As the time for the ceremony draws near, we need to turn our attention away from the external details and prepare ourselves internally for the ritual. This can be particularly hard in a D.I.Y. situation, where the protagonists in the ritual have also taken responsibility for the practical details. It is a little bit like trying to act in a play when we are still thinking about getting the ice creams ready for the interval. Therefore, in the final hours before the ritual, we should delegate roles as much as possible to trusted helpers, in order to be able to bring our attention from the busy periphery of the mind to the quiet centre. If this is not possible, it is best to try to keep the practicalities simple.

Different things help different people to prepare themselves for a ceremony: going for a walk, having a shower or bath, sitting in meditation, doing yoga, or simply spending a quiet moment with the phone off the hook. Not drinking alcohol for at least 24 hours beforehand is generally advisable. Cleansing herbs can also be used just before the ceremony, to bring our own energy field into balance just as we cleansed the room. Ideally this is done by someone else, who wafts the smoke all around you. It is a lovely sensation to be bathed in sweet-smelling herbs, with nothing to do for a moment but breathe in and out.

Some of these preparations can also be built into the ceremony, for the benefit of all the participants. For example: a processional walk, passing around smudge, or just sitting quietly for a few moments together.

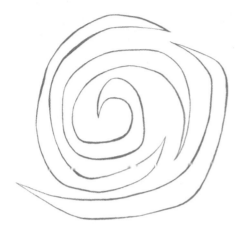

Chapter 3

Devising a Ceremony

Devising a ceremony is probably one part divine inspiration to five parts earthy practicality. On the one hand you will need to meditate on what the ceremony is for, muse on fitting symbols and perhaps browse through books of poetry. On the other hand, you may need to think about parking spaces, access to toilets and what to do if it rains. These humble details are very important. When the practicalities have been well thought out in advance, everyone is comfortable and free to focus on the meaning of the ceremony.

The most important thing is to be clear about the purpose of the ceremony, so the first essential question to ask is: "What are we here to do?" Once that is clear, a time needs to be set aside, and a venue found, bearing in mind the needs of the people you most want to be there. Choosing a time and a place makes the frame for the ceremony. From that point on, the creative process tends to have a will of its own, and I have learnt to trust that the unknown things will become clear in time.

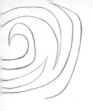

Often, when we ask ourselves a question, we are surprised to find how much we already know. Here are some questions to help you think and plan. Since all the details have a bearing on one another, there is no particular order in which to approach these issues.

What

What is the main intention of the ceremony?

Is there an image that occurs to us when we think about this intention?

Is there anything that we know needs to be included?

Are there any other reasons for the ceremony as well aside from central intention?

What are the emotions surrounding this intention that are likely to need space in the ceremony?

Who

Who are the people we most want to be present?

What do they need in order to be comfortable physically?

What faiths / cultural sensibilities do they come with?

What do they need in order to feel comfortable with the content of the ceremony?

Do any of them have / need a particular role?

Do we want children to be present? If so, how can we make them welcome? If not, do we need to provide a space for them elsewhere so that they don't disrupt the event?

How

Do we want to conduct the ceremony ourselves or ask someone else to lead it?

If the latter, do we want to find a professional celebrant (see list of celebrants at back of book) or is there someone else we know who could hold the space?

Have we heard of any other inspiring events we could borrow from?

How will we inspire our minds and raise our spirits during this ceremony (words, poems, prayers, meditations)?

How will we please and nourish our senses (images, scents, music, flavours, textures)?

How can we involve people of all ages?

When

How soon feels right?

Is the season important?

What time of day?

What meals might be included?

Where

Where do we feel safe, comfortable and uplifted?

Outdoors / indoors?

Access – is it easy to get to for those we want to be present?

Toilets – are there enough? Are they accessible? Do we need to bring some in?

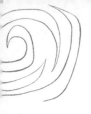

Wet weather options?
Do we need permission?

Details

What clothes help us to feel special, calm and relaxed in ourselves?
Are there any pieces of clothing or jewellery that we might want to wear to remind us of loved ones who may or may not be present?
What food most supports the intention of our ceremony?
Is there a central image or idea that could be represented on the invitations and in the decorations for the space?

How much

How much money does it feel right to spend on this event?
What is our upper limit?

* * *

Finally, a few general tips:

◊ Keep it simple – when an idea reveals itself as simple and obvious, it has matured. The simpler the form, the more you can focus on what you're doing, rather than the stage management.

◊ Be comfortable – take care of everyone's needs to be warm, dry and comfortable, then everyone can relax and be present.

◊ Be inclusive – think about how to make everyone feel welcome. Explaining what you are doing and why can make a big difference to those who aren't used to working in this way. Choose prayers that are open, or explicitly welcome everyone's guides, gods or doubts.

◊ Be imaginative – there are as many different ways to make a ceremony as there are people, so choose something that appeals to your imagination.

◊ Ask for help – many people will respond gladly to being given a role in a ceremony, and this reduces your workload. As well as practical help, you may need emotional support. You can ask for this too!

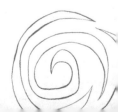

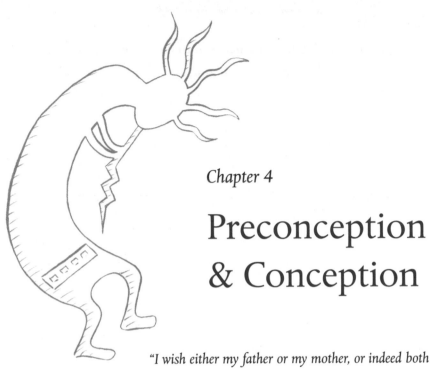

Chapter 4

Preconception & Conception

*"I wish either my father or my mother, or indeed both
of them, as they were in duty both equally bound to it,
had minded what they were about when they begot me."*
L. Sterne 1767

Having a child is a profound change in status and responsibility. It changes your life more dramatically than leaving home, more than starting a relationship or getting married. And although it's completely ordinary, making a new human being is perhaps the most remarkable thing you might do in your life. Giving birth itself is the climax of a long rite of passage that begins with the dance of fertility, the twinkle in the eye. So, when possible, making preparations for this awesome transformation can begin before conception, with a period of purification. It's also joyful to make conscious the request to the universe for the gift of a child. Our ancestors made pilgrimages, wore amulets and bathed in sacred springs to enhance their fertility. Perhaps surprisingly, in our current age of reason, you don't have to travel too far before you find couples following in their footsteps a little, making something sacred of the dance between the man and the woman, the magic of two becoming three.

Purification

Before any ritual, it is common practice to cleanse the space where the ceremony will take place. In this case, the space that is to be cleansed is the body and being of the man and woman themselves. It's easy to see that a foetus thrives best in a living environment free from toxins such as alcohol, cigarette smoke and other poisons. But the mental and emotional state of both mother and father also have an impact on the child, and on the parents' ability to conceive. To understand this better, we could learn from a tradition in Burkina Faso, where a man or woman who is planning to start a family must return to the place of their birth, and if possible the exact tree where their placenta was buried. This is a pilgrimage to revisit the vulnerability of being a child, to honour the parents, and particularly to pray for healing and forgiveness for any hurts received in these early years.[4] There is a great wisdom in this journey. As parents, we are very affected by the kind of treatment we received as children, for good or ill. Becoming conscious of our early experiences gives us more of a chance to choose what we pass on to the next generation, and what we can release and heal. In our culture of geographically dispersed families,

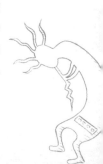

19

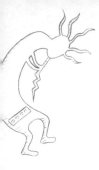

it might not be practical to return to the place of your birth, but the journey to honour your parents and remember your childhood can also be made through an act of creative imagination.

While I was on retreat, preparing to be a mother (although in fact a long way off becoming one), this is a ritual that was suggested to me. Since I had lost both my parents at an early age, the act of visiting them had to be a symbolic one.

I found a quiet spot in the land and made a pile of stones for my mother. I chose things that reminded me of her for one reason or another – a round stone because she was cuddly, a piece of granite for her determination and so on. I talked to her about what I had appreciated about her, and what I was grateful for. I talked to her about my sadness that she couldn't be there with me now, about the disappointment I felt that she had never met my husband, and would never know my children – if I had any. Sometimes I asked questions too, and odd as it may sound, I felt I did understand some answers. It was as if a little part of me had to ask the question, but somewhere a wiser part of me already knew the answers.

I noticed that the pile of stones made for my mother looked very vulnerable and sad. I went in search of something to represent my father. I found a branch with a bend in it, rather like a crooked elbow, and had a strong instinct to put it around the stones so that it held and protected them. I talked to my father. I was very angry that he had not been there for my mother and me all my life. I allowed myself to imagine what I might have been able to share if he had been alive, and asked him over and over why he had to go. I had the strong sense that he was sorry too, that the branch showed what he would have liked to be able to do.

I felt closer to both my mother and father after this. Of course it didn't sort out all the issues once and for all. Years later, I am still grappling with how the losses affect my life, but I think the ritual did start some process of calling things into consciousness, and begin the preparation for parenthood.

I imagine that this exercise could be powerful and transforming even if one's parents were alive. If there are step-parents, adoptive parents or others who played an important role in your early life, they can be included. If you plan to do something along these lines, make sure that are in a safe place where you won't be disturbed, and that you have cleared enough time. This is deep reflective work and may bring up strong feelings, so it is best if you can have some quiet time beforehand and afterwards. It could also help to have a supportive friend to talk to, or even to witness the ritual.

Preparing to conceive a child is also a time when unresolved issues about previous pregnancies are likely to come up. It is as if the womb remembers its past experiences and these may need to be cleansed in some way before it is ready to receive another child. (See also Chapters 10 and 13 on rituals for Miscarriage and Terminating a Pregnancy.)

Michelle: "During the time before conceiving our first child, I was with friends at Christmas. We were talking about children, and I suddenly started crying. I realised it was about a termination I had had ten years ago when I was 22. At that time, I was very clear that I didn't want to have the child, but I didn't think about the enormity of what I was doing. After the termination I felt a kind of hollowness, and for years I was low. My friend suggested I did a little ritual for the child. I just did it quietly in a sitting meditation. I created a space in

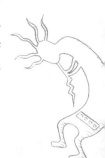

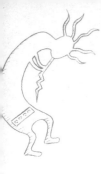

my heart for the child and I talked to it. I said I was sorry I couldn't be there for it at that time, that I would always love this child, and that it would have a place in my heart for as long as it wanted it. For all this time I had been feeling guilty, and at last I set it down. That was just months before John and I conceived."

In Michelle's case, the emotional memory arose spontaneously and she dealt with it quietly and internally, but it is not always easy to access the blockages that hold us back. Visiting a healer or bodyworker is one way to give yourself a chance to heal any unfinished business before conceiving. Maya Abdominal Massage, a traditional discipline from Central America which is becoming available in this country, is particularly good for healing and preparing the woman's reproductive system for conception.[5] (For more on removing blocks to conception, see Chapter 5 on Infertility.)

Invoking Fertility

"Whatever happens here on earth must first be dreamed" Navajo saying

Apart from taking care of our physical, emotional and mental well-being, we can take a further step to declare our readiness to invite a new energy into our lives. In our times, most people have been controlling their fertility for many years before they decide to allow nature to take its course. It can be quite a long journey for a modern man or woman to identify with a positive model of fertility. Images in the media glamourise the youthful body and the independent lifestyle, sex is celebrated in a way that disassociates it from procreation, and rarely do we hear a voice that honours the huge contribution of parents, or indeed the marvel of nature's capacity to create life. Our ancestors had a very different point of view. Here is a piece of erotic poetry from a 4,000-year-old agrarian society in ancient Mesopotamia, where the metaphorical connection between the sacred marriage of the Queen and King and the fertility of the land is explicit.[6]

Inanna spoke:
    "My vulva, the horn,
    The Boat of Heaven,
    Is full of eagerness like the young moon.
    My untilled land lies fallow.
    As for me, Inanna,
    Who will plough my vulva! Who will plough my high field!
    Who will plough my wet ground!"
Dumuzi replied:
    "Great Lady, the king will plough your vulva.
    I, Dumuzi the King, will plough your vulva."
Inanna:
    "Then plough my vulva, man of my heart!
    Plough my vulva!"

At the king's lap stood the rising cedar.
Plants grew high by their side.
Grains grew high by their side.
Gardens flourished luxuriantly.

Invoking fertility is about tuning in to this joyful celebration of sex as divine creativity, believing in the capacity of your body to do this awesome thing, and also about making a direct request to the universe for the blessing of a child. Even though we now know what

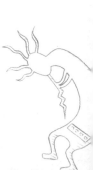

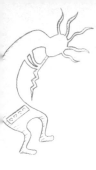

must happen biologically for a healthy embryo to form and implant, walking in our ancestors' footsteps is a way to open ourselves to the dream of welcoming a child into the world, and of offering ourselves as parents.

Making a pilgrimage is one way to express willingness to travel the path of childbearing. Britain is a land rich with places where people have gone for centuries to pray for luck in childbirth. Some people go to a holy well or spring, and wash in the waters. Others go to a cave, and sit within the sacred womb of the earth. Perhaps you know a place in the land that's sacred to you because of your own associations with it. In any of these places you could spend a little time playing with leaves, flowers or stones, making an earth picture as a form of meditation. The ancient Celtic way is to bring an offering to the land, which could be something from your garden, some bread, or a nip of whisky poured onto the ground. (If you bring an offering of this kind, make sure it is going to biodegrade harmoniously with the land, or offer a tasty snack to passing wildlife.) If you have brought nothing with you, but want to leave something of yourself, a hair from your head, tied around a twig, can be your prayer.

For a more home-based invocation, you could collect objects or images that express fertility, and keep them in a pocket or a special bowl or make them into jewellery. Cowry shells, with their natural vulva shape are an obvious choice.[7] Stag's horn, nuts and seedpods celebrate virility in the male. These things can be given as gifts between lovers, to sweeten the flirting with renewed purpose.

Alternatively, you might find inspiration from picture postcards or statues of fertility Gods and Goddesses. One such character is

Kokopeli, a symbol of fertility from the ancient Anasazi civilisation of the American Southwest, who is undergoing something of a revival in the States today. Depicted in rock paintings dating from at least 1000 years ago, Kokopeli plays the flute, carries a sack containing seeds on his back and is usually shown with an erect penis. He is connected with the heat of the earth that warms the ground in preparation for spring planting. Wandering minstrel and merry prankster, Kokopeli is welcomed wherever he goes, bringing rain to make the crops grow, and leaving the women of the village pregnant.

A powerful image of feminine fertility is the Sheela-na-Gig, which dates back to the early Christian Celtic church in Britain and Ireland. Up until the mid sixteenth century, there was a custom of carving images of female figures with accentuated vulvas over the main entrance of churches or castles. Usually the woman is wide-legged and holding open the lips of her vagina to reveal the opening. The name Sheela seems to relate both to the Irish *Sile*, meaning femininity, or an old woman, and *Sidhe* (pronounced *Shee*) meaning a spirit or faery. Whilst some have tried to argue that the image was placed at the door of the church as a warning against the sins of the flesh, older evidence suggests rather that these were highly regarded images, thought to have the power to deflect evil, and symbolic of life, death and regeneration. The dust from rubbing the vulva was also thought to have magical powers of healing and fertility, and evidence of this practice can be seen on some of the Sheelas, especially in Ireland.

Some people have found that the use of words brought their wish for conception clearly into focus:

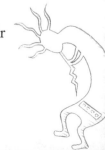

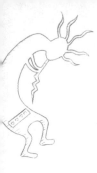

Jane: "We had been keen to conceive as soon as we were married. After two or three months of it not happening, I decided to direct a request to the Great Whoever's Listening. I was at a girlfriend's house. We made a fire and I just wrote a little note saying, "I welcome to the world a healthy happy child for Toby and Jane of 14 Beech Road" and burnt it in the fire. Although I had been open to conceiving before, this brought me to a point of willingness. It brought it into the light. I got pregnant the next month."

One modern Jewish prayer for conception includes a pledge to 'Tikkun Olam' – making the world a more perfect place. The couple give money to charity as a symbol of the work they are committed to 'to make this world worthy of a new presence'. The prayer ends with the words: "Let us now call down the Holy sparks of divinity to join our union in creating a new life." [8]

Elaine: "There were definitely times when I was silently sending up a prayer to a soul, saying 'YES, come on in!' I remember being at a gig. The band were playing this glorious song and my heart was just open, feeling that there was someone there, looking down on me, waiting for the right moment to come in."

Thomas: "The second time we had unprotected sex I invited a being in verbally. There was a sense, an idea, of spirit somehow joining matter. Normally I'm profoundly sceptical. I just don't know whether there is such a thing as a soul or spirit. It was a sort of intuition. But that was definitely the time my wife got pregnant."

It is normal in our culture to be secretive about plans to conceive a child. Yet this position can leave you feeling isolated. If you are offering your home, heart and womb to hold a child, you too may need to feel 'held' by people around you. You can ask people to hold you in mind or pray for you as you prepare to conceive. Sometimes a grandparent feels moved to help on a spiritual level. One woman whose daughter was taking some time to conceive, expressed her support by making a small doll and creating a nest for it in a box. She kept this talisman in a cupboard (unbeknown to the daughter), and her daughter conceived soon afterwards. Perhaps sometimes a soul seeking incarnation is looking for a little more support in the world than a nuclear family or single parent may be able to offer.

* * *

Whilst I do heartily recommend giving some thought to pre-pregnancy preparation, I know that many of us, if we stopped to think too much about having a child, might never do it. With our second child, Phil and I agreed to stop using contraception, but didn't do anything positive to invite a being in. Knowing the reality of looking after one baby, we were pretty daunted about the possibility of having another. She just snuck in when we weren't looking, and is none the less adored.

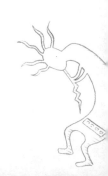

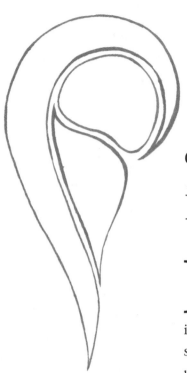

Chapter 5

Infertility

However much we prepare and do our best to make it happen, conception doesn't always come when we want it to. Longing for a child is such a vulnerable state to be in. There is a willingness to love unrequitedly, a great opening of oneself to the possibility of harbouring a child, and yet there is no guarantee that one will come. There are few comparable situations in modern life. We are used to having a measure of control over our environment, our career, even our relationships. Yet in the area of conception, which will probably have the greatest impact on our lives, we are powerless to make anything happen.

I know a little about this misery, because I spent two and a half years in my early thirties trying to conceive before suddenly getting divorced. Years, and many tears later, and with a new partner, it still took over 12 months of anxious waiting. But for some people, what I experienced is merely the prelude to a host of medical tests, difficult decisions and invasive interventions, which may or may not lead to a successful pregnancy.

Some couples conceive one or more children, but then wait years for an addition to their family, which never comes. Secondary infertility can be just as painful and consuming for the parents, added to which they may feel ashamed about their grief, and feel that they should be grateful for what they have.

This is certainly a tough path to tread, a far cry from the climactic conceptions of our dreams. And yet, if we travel prayerfully, with honest searching for what might be blocking a pregnancy, we may find that we are in the end grateful for the way things turned out. We may have had a little more time to do other things and learn more as we ripen.

There are rituals here to help with the waiting period and to take care of yourself if you have to undergo medical tests or treatments. There are stories of those who managed to stay in touch with a sense of a sacred incarnation despite many obstacles, and took their prayers right into the hospital, finding blessing in the miracles that medicine can bring about. And there are suggestions for rituals to lay to rest the dream of a biological family, and make space either for a future without children, or for one open to the possibility of adopting or fostering.

Blocks to Fertility

If conception doesn't happen easily, it is tempting to jump to the conclusion that there is some physical problem with one of the partners. There may be, and fertility clinics are sometimes able to

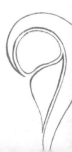

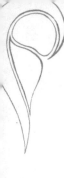

find the physical reason and treat it, but perhaps in pathologising the situation we miss an opportunity to access a greater wisdom: why is the body saying no? A conception is something that mysteriously involves three people, embedded in an environment that affects each of them cell by cell. There are subtle forces at play here; conception is age-old, but it is delicate. One of the tasks of this life-stage, then, is honestly wondering: what might I need to shift to become ready? This is a question you can be asking whether or not you are also engaging with fertility tests and even treatments.

Maybe the body isn't ready. It may be as simple, and as intractable, as one of the couple needing to give up smoking. Or there may be other invisible toxins or nutritional deficiencies to blame. An organisation called Foresight has developed a comprehensive pre-conception programme which aims for optimal health in both partners, to increase their chances of producing strong sperm and ova. The programme, lasting 4-6 months, requires both to adopt an excellent diet with an emphasis on organic foods and filtered water, and to refrain from alcohol, cigarettes and street drugs. Laboratory analysis of hair is used to check an individual's levels of vitamins, minerals, toxic metals and essential trace elements. Based on these results, an individual regime of cleansing toxins and supplementary nutrients is prescribed. Genito-urinary infections, parasites and allergies are all investigated and treated if found. Foresight claims a high level of success in assisting couples to conceive healthy babies without IVF. Some couples who have opted for IVF have also followed the Foresight plan to give their implanted embryos the best chance. One couple, who had given up on ever having children, decided to follow the Foresight programme as a way of repairing the damage done by years of fertility drugs. After two months they conceived naturally.

Sometimes stress is a contributing factor and one or both of the couple needs to slow down, or perhaps find a different job. Pregnancy is a taxing state for a woman's body, and if she is depleted energetically, her body may reasonably decide to keep its resources to itself. This could be your body's call to allow yourself some therapeutic input, such as Maya Abdominal Massage, Shiatsu, Acupuncture or Cranial Sacral Therapy. [9]

A holistic treatment like one of these might also be able to identify and shift an emotional block. After nearly a year of failing to conceive with my second husband I went to see a healer who scanned my aura. What she saw was a great deal of fear constraining my creativity. When she asked me to speak about it, out tumbled a host of fears about how having a child would wreck my life and leave me exhausted, with no space for my other loves: music and writing. Her spiritual guide gave me great reassurance that all would be well. I can't say that I understand what she saw, or how she dealt with it, but the very next month I conceived.

Or perhaps it really isn't the right time, place, or even partner. With hindsight I can see that at the time I was praying hard for a child with my first husband, it was as well that my prayers were denied.

A Meditation for Women waiting for Conception

Waiting to conceive, if it goes on a long time, can be very straining, especially for women. Month by month we begin with hope and excitement, obsessively watching for signs that this month the cycle

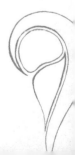

31

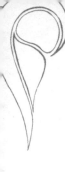

will be different, only to come up against disappointment and grief at the first feeling of an all-too familiar heaviness, the first showing of blood. If not addressed, these feelings can harden into a sense of failure, a lack of faith in the body, or a consuming anger that the world is not as we would have it. Apart from anything else, none of these states of mind are likely to lead to more frequent love-making, which has to be top of the 'things to do' list when trying to make a baby.

I offer here a two-part meditation to support women waiting to conceive. It uses a bowing practise, adapted from the Sufi way of prayer, which involves coordinating the breath with simple movements of the body. The beauty of this practise is that it can take us beyond the busy mind to listen to the whispers or the soul. At the beginning of the monthly cycle, it is a quest for an answer to the question: "What must I do to be ready to conceive?" If conception doesn't happen, it is an opportunity to process the feelings that arise. It acts as an antidote to bitterness and initiates a search for gratitude for what is nevertheless good in our lives.

You will need a white cloth and a white candle, a red cloth and a red candle.

Find a little place in your house to set up an altar that you can sit before. Use the white cloth and white candle, together with any other objects or pictures that appeal to you, to make an altar to your own fertility. If you are using a thermometer or other means to keep track of or enhance your fertility, you could keep these things on the altar too.

Light the candle and settle into silence. As you breathe, send your awareness around your body, paying special attention to your mind, heart and womb.

Opening Prayer: Great Mother, you know all about circles and cycles. You know the longing in my heart to conceive a child. This month I offer my womb to be a nesting place for a new life. I feel … (Allow space to name any feelings that come up, but don't spend longer than 5 minutes on this.) I ask for guidance in my meditation today.

Bowing Practise: sitting or kneeling, take a breath in. As you breathe out, bow forward, taking your forehead towards the floor as far as is comfortable. Take the question, "What must I do to be ready to conceive a child?" deep into your heart, deep into your belly, all the way to the earth. Rest a moment between breaths, at the bottom, in the place of unknowing. Breathe in as you rise again, being sensitive to any answers that may come. Some people see images, others hear words or simply know things. Breathe out and let the impact of the answer, if any, ripple through you. Begin again, or rest for a few breaths at the top if you need to. Carry on for as long as it is fruitful. Whatever comes up, be it an answer you like or don't like, or no answer at all, plough this back into the next bow and send it to the earth for healing. Finally, rest and contemplate any wisdom you have received.

If the breathing and bowing is difficult or uncomfortable for you, you could lie or sit instead and visualise taking your question to a wise and beneficent being.

Closing Prayer: Compassionate Mother, thank you for your guidance. Bless our lovemaking this month, and may your will be done. I pray for patience and I surrender to your perfect timing.

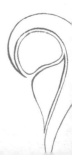

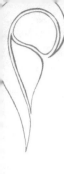

If this month does not bring a pregnancy, and the blood starts to come, put away the objects from the white altar and keep them in a safe place. Make a new altar using the red cloth and red candle, together with any other objects or pictures that speak to you of your passionate life as a woman (not just a mother); aspects of your life that will benefit from increased energy and time if you are not pregnant or looking after a baby.

Light the red candle and settle into silence. As you breathe, send your awareness around your body, paying special attention again to your mind, heart and womb.

Opening Prayer: Great Mother, I sit here knowing that this month no child is coming to our family. My heart is sad because I wanted to have a baby. I feel … (Make space for any feelings that come up, but again not more than 5 minutes). Bless me and hold me during the time of my bleeding.

Bowing Practise: This time there is a circling of the head before the bow. Breathing in, circle your head over your left shoulder, round the front with your chin to your chest and back over your right shoulder. As you do this, imagine that you are gathering up all your riches into a basket, everything you have to be thankful for in your life as it is now. Breathe out as you bow and bring your treasure to the earth, giving thanks. As you breathe in, rise up with your empty basket. Breathe out at the top and place your hands open, palms up, ready to receive. Continue circling and bowing, letting other things come into your basket as they occur to you, resting in openness, with faith in the world to bring you good things. You may find that ingratitude and anger arise when you do this exercise – inevitably, for each quality brings with it its opposite. If this happens, gather up your feelings and plough them back into your bowing practise, bringing these to the earth too for healing. This is a crucial part of an authentic practise, and in the eyes of the Divine Mother is simply very human.

Closing Prayer: Bless me as a woman in my life as it is. May this be a time of healing and acceptance.

At the end of your period, put away the objects from the red altar, and when you feel ready, lay out the white altar again.

When going to the Doctor or Hospital for Tests

No-one wants to talk to doctors about their sex life, far less be poked and prodded, asked to produce a sperm sample on demand, or submit to a stranger's enquiring latex-gloved hand. This kind of violation is apt to make a sensitive person's sex drive flee to a distant hiding place.

If you have to go to the doctor for tests, try to take a moment to check in with yourself beforehand. It's best to do this at home if possible, but you could do it whilst sitting in the waiting room, if need be. Breathe gently and send your awareness to the part of your body that's about to be examined. See if you can feel any sensation there. Imagine sending your breath to this area. Visualise a warm and vibrant light in your sexual organs, as a way of giving them protection and love. After the examination, do the same, giving yourself time to feel and release any tensions.

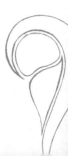

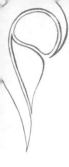

When you next come to have sex, you may need extra sensitivity to coax you gently back into sensuality, and it might be as well to ask your partner to be prepared for some tears along the way.

Rituals during Fertility Treatments

Even, or perhaps especially, when the sacred mystery of conception becomes a medical procedure, we need prayer and ritual to counter-balance the starkness of such interventions.

I talked to Alan, a woodsman, who, after a series of hospital tests, was told that his sperm was infertile due to a congenital disease, affecting one in a thousand men. It was a terrible shock for both him and his wife, Zara.

Alan: "It's really unfair, but I started to see parallels in nature. 30% of a tree's seed will be infertile. Nettles don't produce much fertile seed; they spread by cloning. I'm lucky that my wife was supportive of trying to conceive with donated sperm. The most important thing for us was to create new life together, not to have our own baby. I can't have my own genetic child, but it doesn't mean I'm impotent. My potency and potential is in making the wild places beautiful. It's made me more focussed on what I want to do in the world."

Before conception Alan and his wife went to the 'ladywell' near where they lived; a place that's been associated with fertility for about 1,000 years. Zara bathed in the water. After each insemination, Alan and Zara went to sit under an oak tree together in the hospital grounds. Whilst it was far from what they had wanted in terms of how their children were conceived, this was at least something they could do together to reclaim their sense of the sacred.

If we are bold, we can take our ritual right into the medical establishment itself. Here is a Rabbi's story, which shows how someone working within their tradition can draw on well-known prayers and bring them into a modern application.[10]

"On the day that our clinically fertilised embryos were due to be placed in my partner's womb, we arrived at the doctor's office and were sent to a small procedure room. After details and paper work, my wife lay down in the hospital bed and the medical staff left us alone. I stood at the foot of the bed and recited the afternoon prayer. Afterwards, we held hands and talked about the life that we wanted to create. We invited God to send a soul that was compassionate, vivacious, and loving to animate the cells that would soon be slipped into my wife's body. We shifted our attention away from the fog of medical technology and stopped to appreciate the yearning call of creation that enveloped us. Finally, we said this blessing from the wedding ceremony together:

'We stand in awe of Your blessings, our God, for creating man and woman in Your image, and blessing them with the power to create new life. Bless you, God, for creating human life.'

Our ritual closed with a kiss. Then the staff arrived in sterile scrubs. That was fine. This time God had arrived first."

Accepting Infertility

Longing to conceive a child and feeling thrilled in case this month will be the one, followed by crashing disappointment when it isn't, all takes up a great deal of one's physical and emotional resources. There may come a time when enough is enough and, for whatever

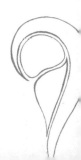

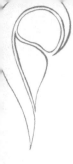

reason, we call a halt to the dream of conceiving. It may be that a physical transition, such as moving house, marks the change.

Abbey: "After our third miscarriage, Andrew said he didn't want to try again. It was time to let go, and it felt like a good thing. I've recently moved from that house to a new flat. The house was a rambling place, with lodgers, and it would have been big enough for a family. Moving to this new flat feels like entering a different era. We had buried our third miscarried foetus in the garden and planted a bush on top. We left the bush there for other people to enjoy the beauty and the blossoms without knowing its history, and that feels right."

If something external like this doesn't take place, then the decision, although momentous, is an event without a landmark. Ending unsuccessful fertility treatment, or deciding not to try again after a series of miscarriages is not something that one actively 'does', so much as stops doing. In these circumstances doing something symbolic to close the possibility, actively and definitely, helps us to regain some power in an area where we can feel very out of control.

For someone who is thinking of adopting a child, acknowledging the disappointment of not being a biological parent, of not passing on the ancestral line, is important preparation. Having done this, we are freer to accept the joys and responsibility of receiving someone else's child into our home. (For more on this subject, see Chapter 12.)

I offer here a simple ritual, which can be adapted as necessary. It is focussed on a practical clearout of your house, which is useful in itself, and also represents an inner process of clearing space for good new things.

The Ritual

You could do this work alone, but it is strongly recommended that you work with your partner and / or ask one or two close friends to be supportive witnesses.

You will need one large candle and about a dozen night-lights.

Preparation

Go through your house room by room and gather together any evidence of your longing for a child (or another child). This could be anything you may have collected or kept, consciously or unconsciously, like a pram in the loft, baby clothes or books you were saving for future children. It might be paraphernalia to do with checking fertility, letters from a fertility clinic, or fertility-enhancing herbs you've been taking.

When you are ready to proceed to the next part, prepare a space to be clean and free from disturbances. Set out all the objects you have gathered together on a cloth in the centre of the room.

Opening Meditation

Sit quietly near the objects with eyes closed, and let your mind settle until you are aware of your breath. Pay particular attention to the sensations arising in your heart and your womb. Imagine a person or a circle of people with you who love and support you. These could be loved ones or spiritual mentors in your real life, or an imagined guide.

When you are ready, open your eyes and look at the objects in front of you. Give yourself time to feel the impact of seeing these things out in the open, and say whatever comes up to be said. Now look through the objects you have collected and decide what to do

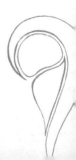

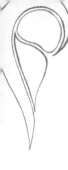

with each of them. Some could perhaps be passed on to friends or a charity shop; some could carefully disposed of. Some might be kept for visiting children to enjoy. Ask for practical help from your witnesses. If there is more stuff than you can deal with now, just do a little and make a firm intention to clear it out by a certain time – whatever is reasonable for you. For now, move all the items out of the room you're working in. If this isn't possible, move them to the edge of the room and put them in a bag or cover with a cloth. There should now be a space in the middle of the room.

Cleansing
Pass around a bowl of water and a towel so that everyone can wash their hands. Take as long as you need, as this is a symbolic act of moving from one state to another.

New Dreams
In the centre of your clear space, light a candle to represent new hopes and dreams that can enter the space. From this flame, you might like to light night-lights and state particular new things that you commit to letting into your life, new ways to be potent, creative and nurturing. Or you could ask your witnesses to do this for you, making wishes on your behalf. Keep the central candle after the ceremony, and burn it to help remind you of promises made to yourself.

Closing Meditation
Either close your eyes or focus gently on the burning candles. Breathe deeply and pay attention to the sensations arising now in your body, particularly in the heart and womb areas. Notice if anything is different from when you began. Remember the guides

you called on at the beginning, thank them and let them go. When you are ready to finish, signal the end of the meditation, and close by sharing warming food and drink, whilst enjoying the candlelight.

This is a ritual for an early stage of accepting infertility. Later on, you might want to look at Chapter 14 on Not Having Children, for suggestions of more ways to affirm your creativity and potency in the world.

A Memorial Service

The above ritual is something that can be carried out as an individual, supported by a friend or partner. However, given that fertility issues are often kept secret, it can be particularly healing to be part of a group of others who understand your losses.

Members of the British Infertility Counselling Association used to run an annual non-denominational service for people to acknowl-edge losses associated with infertility, failed fertility treatment, lost pregnancies or unwanted childlessness for any reason. The service was run by volunteers, all of whom had themselves experienced fertility losses, and was designed to reach out to people of all faiths or none.

Amongst readings and participative prayers, people were invited to light a candle for those children who were not in life (even those who were never physically conceived). A large bouquet of colourful flowers was placed in the centre of the room, and people were encouraged to cut a blossom representing their lost child and float it in a bowl of water. Time was set aside for people to write messages

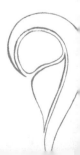

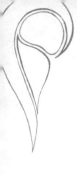

to these missing children, and the messages were ritually burnt after the end of the service. A pebble was also provided for each person, as a symbol of the burdens picked up along the fertility path, the weight that sometimes settles in the heart or the stomach. People could write or draw on the pebble and leave it on the central table to be released back to the sea following the service.

The final prayer was as follows:

"Creator of all Life, we believe your love for all children is strong and enduring. We were not able to know our children as we'd hoped. May our hearts be opened by our experiences, not closed. We offer thanks for family, friends and counsellors who have supported and encouraged us in times of need. We remember all who suffer losses similar to ours, particularly those who haven't had the same opportunity for support. We pray for the staff at hospitals and clinics. Help them to learn and advance in all their work. We offer thanks for all living children and pray especially for those in any need. Give us all courage to face the future, whatever it holds. Help us transform our experiences into wisdom and compassion for everything that lives. Hear us now in silent prayer."

The service provided healing and comfort to many, and is still held from time to time, although, at the time of writing, no longer on an annual basis. You can find more information from the British Infertility Counselling Association (see p.185) or request a copy of the full text of the ceremony from Meredith Wheeler (see p.188).

* * *

We may call for the blessing of children and be denied it, and yet we may find creativity flowing into our lives in other ways. Kokopeli, that ancient one with his seed sack and his flute, is the bringer not just of children but also of music and joy. Ultimately, our appreciation of fertility cannot be limited to whether or not we have children. It is about celebrating all the ways in which human beings can conceive ideas, cross-fertilize productively and generate beauty. It is about appreciating the verdant earth, which burgeons irrepressibly each spring, and of which we are a living part. And, it is a journey that can bring us to the heart of our vulnerability, teaching us to live with the struggle of wanting something passionately in the face of our own limitations to make it happen.

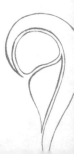

Chapter 6

Pregnancy

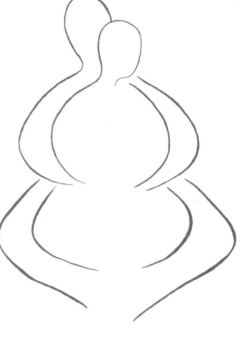

"*Dancing,*
I am dancing inside!
Two pink lines,
One fainter than the other,
But two
Pink
Lines!
And you, with a dreamy look,
Taking it in,
Smile lines creasing around your eyes.
I am so glad."

J Singer 2005

Some people have a sense right from conception that a child has been formed, or are lucky enough to have a numinous dream, such as a door opening and light coming through. For the rest of us, the herald of this momentous change is a general physical malaise, as the body succumbs to the dramatically different instructions given by a new cocktail of hormones. In my own case,

I felt constipated, exhausted, and inexplicably miserable for quite a few days, before it occurred to me what the physical cause for feeling all at sea might be. Then there is the moment of truth, not just an absence of blood in its due time, but the definite presence of a little line in a viewing window of the pregnancy test. In our age this is a profound moment: the first outward sign of an invisible new reality.

A positive pregnancy test may prompt a wide range of emotional responses. Yet even if the initial feeling is wonder and delight, this seems to come hand in hand with a host of fears and anxieties. What if I lose the baby? What if I don't – will I be able to cope? Where will we live? How will we make ends meet? What about my job / career / travel plans / body image / independent lifestyle?

The inner work of pregnancy is that of keeping pace with the journey that our body is taking us on, whether it is a straightforward development of a healthy baby or a pregnancy full of physical complications and emotional strain. Even when there is great joy at the start of a pregnancy, it is a time of sacrifice for a woman too, as she begins to let go of some of the freedoms she has been used to and literally surrenders her body to the demands of another person. And with all the changes coming so fast, it is a time of vulnerability, when a woman needs a great deal of holding. Perhaps some of this vulnerability is actually the experience of the child, finding itself on a new and bemusing plane, and needing reassurance that this is a good place to be.

On the other hand, pregnancy is a very special time spiritually. Women seem to experience the world from a much more inner place than usual, when they are carrying a child. There is a natural inclination to withdraw from the world, to move at a slower pace

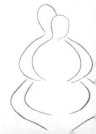

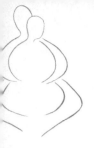

and with a stiller mind, closer to meditation. For all the physical aches and pains, pregnancy can be a state of grace, when a woman is at her most radiant.

Antenatal care in our culture, based at the doctor's surgery and maternity hospital, is very good at picking up problems and spotting abnormalities in pregnancy, but hardly touches on the wider emotional and spiritual story told through each individual's experience of bringing a new person into the world. In this chapter I hope to offer a different context in which to frame the experience of pregnancy and preparation for birth, with meditations for different stages of the baby's growth, comparisons from other cultures around the world, and then stories of three different ceremonies created to support and celebrate mothers-to-be as they approach birth and motherhood. The next chapter, on Birth, continues this preparation through the later days of pregnancy, as the arrival of the child draws near.

Meditations for the Early Days

In the very earliest days of my first pregnancy I came across a prayer by St Teresa of Avila, a 16th century Spanish nun, that gave me great comfort. In the midst of a torrent of hormones and emotions, these words seemed to be just what I needed to hear. I put the prayer to a simple tune and sang it to myself often. When my daughter Heather was born I sang it to her too.

Nada te turbe,
nada te espante;
todo se pasa,
Dios no se muda.
La pacientia todo lo alcanza.
Quien a Dios tiene, nada la falta:
solo Dios basta.

Let nothing disturb you,
Let nothing frighten you;
All things pass away,
God* never changes.
Patience obtains all things.
Whoever has God lacks nothing:
God alone suffices.

* You may wish to substitute 'Love' for 'God' if this has more meaning for you.

Meditation to make Contact with the Child

In the first weeks of pregnancy, despite the immediate and dramatic changes to the mother's body, the presence of the new being is very subtle. For myself, during the early uncertain days, I felt that I wanted to reach out to the soul of the child and express a quiet welcome and an invitation to settle in. This seemed in stark contrast to the language of screening and testing – the way of our current antenatal services. I wanted my first communication with the foetus to be, "Hello, welcome!" rather than "Are you normal?". I contacted a doula

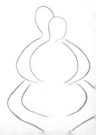

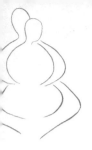

(a birth partner) and was introduced to a different way of making contact with the baby, which was about sensitively communicating rather than objectively 'scanning'. Doulas work alongside midwives to support women emotionally and practically through pregnancy and birth, and I certainly found that involving one offered me a more holistic approach.[11]

This is the meditation that my doula guided me through, and which I was able to use on my own at other times throughout the pregnancy:

Sit comfortably and let your breath settle into a rhythm. Bring your hands to your belly and bring your attention inside to your womb. Speak silently to greet and welcome the baby, and say anything you want about how you feel about its arrival. See the womb as a room and visualise making it ready, just as you would for a guest. Dust the surfaces, add fresh flowers, light a candle, whatever feels right.

Ask your baby if there is anything that he needs to help him come into life and just listen for responses. (You may not hear words, but you might see an image or have an intuitive sense of an answer.) You could ask how he feels about ultrasound or any other tests you are thinking of having. Or use this opportunity to explain if there is something coming up that he needs to prepare for. Later on in pregnancy you can ask if there is anything the baby needs to help prepare for birth. Finish the conversation and return to quiet breathing. Open your eyes when you are ready.

Don't worry if you don't feel you had any clear answers to questions. Sometimes just asking the question can bring about clarity because it acknowledges that the child has a point of view. However, if you do have a strong intuition about a response, be sure to honour it if you can. This builds trust and respect between mother and baby.

Marking the End of the First Trimester

After the first 12 weeks of pregnancy the tiny foetus is fully formed and the pregnancy is much more secure. It is as if a decision has now been made about whether the relationship between mother and child will hold. In our culture this is commonly the time when the secret of the pregnancy is made public. Traditional societies have acknowledged this threshold in more poetic ways. Chinese traditional medicine holds that the 'Shen' (soul) of a child moves in at about three months. This is the point in Acupuncture practice when a special point called 'House Guest' is warmed with a herb, 'moxa', in order to nourish the body deeply. For Australian Aboriginals it is not until a woman feels the first kick from the unborn child that conception is deemed to have taken place. At that moment, a spirit child in the land is believed to have sprung up into her womb and sung the foetus into life.[12]

One thing my partner and I did around this time in my first pregnancy was buy a big candle with three wicks. Lighting one for me, one for him and one for the baby was a simple way to focus our minds on the growing family. We sometimes just sat with him behind me, and the candle in front for a few minutes in silence, taking in the new reality. After such moments we often shared good conversations, which got straight to the heart of things and brought us closer. It was much harder to find time to do this with our second pregnancy, added to which a candle with four wicks seemed to

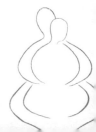

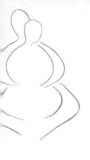

result in lots of leaking wax and mess! Another way to mark the occasion could be to go to a special place in the land and take an offering of thanks, especially if you embarked on a pilgrimage to ask for the blessing of fertility before this pregnancy. Or you could book a massage, or simply have a special dinner and chink a glass to celebrate.

Meditation on Circles of Support

It is not only the mother who feels the need for extra holding during pregnancy; the father too bears a new responsibility, and may well feel a whole fresh set of demands upon him. The following meditation, given to my partner and me by my Sufi teacher, focuses on the need of both parents to be supported as they prepare themselves for parenthood. It can be done at any stage of the pregnancy. You could of course do this on your own, if your partner is absent or unwilling.

Sit opposite each other so that the baby is between you, and hold hands if this is comfortable. Settle for a few minutes as you let your breath find a rhythm, and become aware of each other's breathing. Focus your awareness on your heart and on opening to the heart of your partner. After a while, shift your awareness to the mother's womb and to the baby safely held there between you.

Now visualise behind you the people who are supporting you as you go through this change. Acknowledge your parents and grandparents, whether they are alive or not. Then remember other family members and close friends, and beyond these greater circles of support. Behind all of these you might like to imagine a spiritual presence holding all of the human helpers. You could see it as a guardian angel or a great dove holding out its wings and keeping all under protection.

Sit a little while in the knowledge of this support and practise leaning back into it, as if into an armchair. Have an awareness of all the support behind your partner too, which joins up with yours to form a circle surrounding both of you with love.

When you are ready, return briefly to an awareness in the heart and a steady breathing. Open your eyes when you are ready. If you like, take some coloured pencils or pastels to make a sketch of this image or sensation.

Practical Preparations in the Home

Part of the work of pregnancy is thinking about how to adapt your home for the arrival of a new member of the family. Even this practical task can take on emotional significance. So, here is a little story about interior decorating. During the middle stage of my first pregnancy, I, like many mothers-to-be, was taken over by the nesting instinct, obsessing night and day about storage solutions, the colours of walls, and in particular a pair of beautiful curtains in a fabric I had fallen in love with. I fretted about whether I could afford them, felt sick at the idea of not having them, and eventually worked out a compromise of buying the materials and seeking help to make them myself. In the end, this led to a very satisfying few days of working on my mother's old sewing machine. I felt soothed by the sound of that motor, familiar from childhood, and happy to be in contact with my mother's tools, as I prepared to be a mother myself. Those curtains became emblematic of what I wanted to pass on to

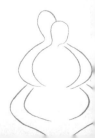

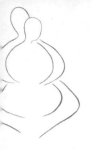

my daughter, something of visual beauty, but also a connection to her ancestors. This is how it is with preparations for our children: the mundane becomes symbolic; the outer expresses the inner.

Mother Blessings

At seven months, or the beginning of the third trimester, the focus of pregnancy begins to shift towards preparations for birth and the arrival of the child. Many traditional societies hold a ceremony at this time.

In Java, the main island of Indonesia, a feast with many symbolic foods is served in the home of the pregnant woman's mother. Rice of three colours is served: red for the father, white for the mother and a mixture of the two to symbolise the child. The midwife who will attend the birth performs a ritual of cutting a leaf in half, while chanting,

> "In the name of God, the Merciful, the Compassionate
> My intention is to cut open a young unopened leaf.
> But I am not cutting open a leaf,
> I am cutting the way open for a baby to emerge.
> I limit you (the baby) to nine months of meditation in your
>   mother's womb.
> Come out easy, go out easy,
> Easy, easy, by the will of Allah"

Sometimes an egg is dropped down the pregnant woman's sarong to make it break, as a symbol of opening up her body for an easy birth.[13]

In the United States, when a birth draws near, a baby shower is announced. Generally, this is a party organised by a close friend of the mom-to-be, and attended by female friends, at which silly games focusing on babies are played (e.g. guess the girth of the mom, guess the flavour of the baby food in unmarked jars) and everyone brings a gift of something that will be needed when the baby is born. Sometimes the father is also involved. While a baby shower is simply a light-hearted party, helping the mother in practical ways to prepare for life with the baby, it also seems to be a modern answer to an age-old call to gather the community around the incoming baby, and support the mother through the birth and beyond.

In recent years, some people have been opting for an alternative baby shower, or 'mother blessing', a ceremony to empower the woman for the challenge of giving birth. This has its roots in something much older than the baby shower: the Blessingway or Beautyway. This is a sacred ceremony conducted by the Navajo people (native to South Western America) to sustain an individual at any critical juncture in his or her life, including a mother before birth. It includes chanting, grooming, gift giving and food sharing, and is a fundamental element of the Navajo way of life. Elements of this ritual have inspired American and British people to create mother blessing ceremonies. (It is important to acknowledge that the Navajo people do not approve the use of the name Blessingway to describe anything other than their own traditional rites.)

A mother blessing ceremony might include some of the following elements:

A gathering of women who have given birth, who may tell their birth stories, or share helpful experiences.

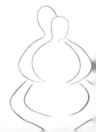

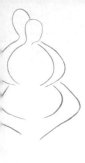

Reflections / prayers / meditations / poems / songs on the theme of the Mother.

Hair brushing, foot washing and / or massage of the mother-to-be. In Navajo tradition, washing the feet is symbolic of preparing for a journey.

The making of something to sustain and encourage the mother in labour, for example a necklace of beads (see below) or a string of prayer flags which can hold the affirmations of the community for the mother in labour.

A celebratory meal, which could include emphasis on round foods (imagine soft loaves of risen bread, ripe pears, mango or melon, Summer pudding etc.)

Gifts of food – each guest brings a nutritious dish that can be kept in the freezer and eaten during the early days after birth, when there may not be time or energy for cooking.

The making of something from the community for the child e.g. a mobile of small gifts, or a quilt made of fabric squares from different people. Distant relatives and friends can send something to be included.

* * *

Here are three stories of women who decided, for quite different reasons, to gather their friends around them as a source of strength during the last term of pregnancy.

Caroline was pregnant with her second child when she read an article by Jeannine Parvati Baker about a Mother Blessing ceremony.

It was described as a way to surround the mother-to-be with gifts of the spirit, and affirm that she will have a natural and beautiful birth experience. Caroline contacted a celebrant she had met in the past, Lu Garner, who agreed to organise it for her.

"The mother blessing was arranged for two weeks before the baby was due. I asked four women friends, so with Lu and I there were just six in total, and they were all mothers. My partner was sceptical about the whole idea, so we gave him the role of looking after our three-year-old son and preparing a feast for afterwards. I felt that it ought to be a women's thing anyway.

When the time came, my blood pressure was steadily going up, and I was being monitored in hospital three days a week. The day before the mother blessing, we had been told by a rather aggressive consultant obstetrician that a home birth was out of the question. Fortunately the community midwives team told us that it was still possible, as long as we were prepared to come into hospital on their advice. I was relieved that I had the party as something positive to focus on. I felt it was about reclaiming my power to give birth naturally and in a place of my own choosing.

Lu came the evening before to prepare the space. We cleansed the living room and transformed the fireplace into a kind of altar with blue and green cloths including a baby sling and towel, shells, candles, and family photographs.

Lu explained what we would do, and led a song and a meditation on the connections between women as mothers across the ages and around the world.

I had asked everyone to bring beads, and as they gave them to me, they gave me a wish, thought or blessing. One by one, I strung the beads onto a necklace to wear during labour. There were times

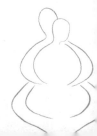

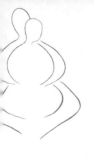

when I couldn't get the needle through, but that was like labour – it took some effort! At one point my son came in, grabbed the necklace and broke it, but that was OK, because it gave me the chance to remake it again a little stronger.

We went into the garden and drank a toast of spring water. Lu anointed me with water on my brow, hands and feet, asking for a graceful birth. Then we poured the water on the earth and asked for her blessings.

We went back up to the house to share gifts, which included poems, songs, a book, some bath oil and a present for Luke. In return I gave everyone a gift of some handmade soap, and a candle, which I hoped they would light for the baby and me as I was giving birth. To finish they made me a garland with flowers from the garden and gave me a foot massage. Lu closed the ceremony and by that time I felt uplifted and ready for anything.

I checked my blood pressure that evening and was pleased to find it was lower than it had been in about three weeks. I sat quietly in the living room, which seemed like a bowl full of calm energy, and went to bed feeling relaxed and strengthened. At about half past three the following morning I awoke to find my waters had broken! I wore the necklace during labour, and at crucial times during contractions when I felt that I couldn't go on, the necklace seemed to brush or bump against my face and remind me that I was not alone. Ciaran was born in the living room at twenty past eight that evening."

* * *

Sian had longed to have a child for years, but when she found she was pregnant she was in the process of splitting up with her partner.

After much agonising, she decided to keep the child, but was understandably anxious about how she would cope on her own.

"The idea of having a 'Community Day' came about because I was pretty sure I would not get any support from the father. I've always believed it's important for a child to grow up with lots of adults in their life, but because of my own situation, I was really looking for reassurance that there would be people I could turn to. Also, because the pregnancy had been such a difficult time emotionally, I hadn't been telling people or even admitting to myself that I was pregnant some of the time. At five months I had in some sense 'come out', but the Community Day, a month before the due date, was another stage of accepting that it was actually going to happen, and saying to my friends, 'There's a new being coming and I want you to be involved.'"

Generally, I don't find asking for help easy, so making an event out of it helped to make it less awkward. It really helped having someone else make flyers and organise it on my behalf.

I wanted there to be lots of people present and there were – 25 or so men, women and children in my living room. It was special to have it in my home (even though it was cramped) because I have the memory of everyone sitting round in a big circle. People were invited to make an offering – a gift, or a poem, or to say some words about their own experience of parenting. Then we went for a walk to the river nearby, and took photos of me with the bump and a bunch of friends around me.

When we came back, we laid out a big sheet of drawing paper and pens, asking people to draw round their hands then write messages of support and their phone numbers. I've mostly forgotten what

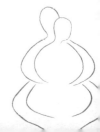

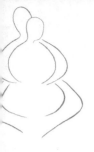

people said when we went round the circle, but what I have got is that piece of paper by the phone. In a blue moment I look at that, and it's a very tangible evidence of a host of aunties and uncles to call upon. At the end of the day, I felt very supported.

In hindsight I think that having the little children in the circle was a mixed blessing. On the one hand, their energy was a reminder of the reality of what was to come – the little ball of chaos inside! But they did demand a lot of our attention. Another time I would suggest that an adult took the children to a next door room to do an activity like making a card for the mother-to-be."

Sian's daughter was born a month later in a birthing pool, and already has many friends in her community.

* * *

My own mother blessing took a different form from either of these. Reflecting on it now, I realise it was not just about preparing for the birth, but also for the life of mothering that followed. I devised the ceremony with a friend, Margot Oakenby, who had plenty of experience with ritual although had not held a mother blessing before. A month before my due date I invited seven women who were all mothers and rather boldly included my partner's mother as one of these. Although we were still getting to know each other, I wanted to invite her into my world and make her feel very welcome as grandmother-to-be. I also invited a friend who I had asked to be present at the birth, which we planned as a home water birth.

We lit a candle and acknowledged my mother's significant absence (because she had died many years earlier), bringing her into the circle by passing around her photograph. Then, as a way of focussing our minds, we asked each woman to speak about the best thing and the hardest thing about being a mother.

Then, we set about making a birth-blessing necklace. I had asked people to bring a bead or charm that could be threaded on a necklace, and the women took turns to present these to me. As it happened, the first woman to come forward brought hers with a song, which we took up as a refrain while I threaded each bead. Her gift was a wooden image of a seal and the lyric to the song was, "O let the motion of the ocean do all of the work." I remember other beads signifying Earth (a stone), Love (a heart), Majesty (a shiny bead like a crown), Flow (a shell from the sea) and Lightness (a little jingly bell and some jesters ribbons to remind me to keep a sense of humour and not aim to be perfect). I threaded some plain black and white beads between the charms, and the whole thing was on a piece of sturdy gold elastic, so it was simple to tie with a knot. When it was complete it looked beautiful and powerful. I looked forward to putting it on when the time came.

Then we went out into the small garden and set up a symbolic journey; this was the idea that Margot and I had come up with for giving shape to the transition I felt I was about to make. Different women took different roles. Behind a curtain of gauzy veils we set a bowl of water with soap and a towel. I started there, with one friend asking me what I was leaving behind. What occurred to me was my independence, my known world, a level of freedom and spontaneity. I spoke about these things and then washed my hands. Meanwhile, women the other side of the veils were softly chanting a Native American song "I walk in beauty, beauty before me, beauty behind me, beauty all around me."

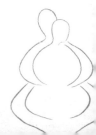

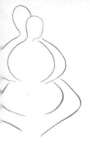

It was time to go through the veils to the other side. The friend who was going to be present at the birth came with me on the journey, but it was up to me to part the veils and push through. I felt a huge amount of fear doing this, which I can't fully explain. Beyond fear of giving birth, or fear of the challenge and responsibility of becoming a mother, I think there was also fear of coming into the world more fully myself, of really being seen for who I am. Perhaps there was a release of fear from the baby I was before my own birth. Who knows if there was an element of my baby's anxiety about being born too. Whatever, it took me quite a long time, with much trembling and many tears to get through! On the other side I was greeted by a little corridor of singing, dancing women, and at the end of that I was draped with a special cloth, handed a bouquet of garden blooms and crowned with a garland of flowers. I needed to stamp and dance to ground my rather wobbly energy at that point. Then we came indoors and I sat while people surrounded me, laid a hand on me and sang a lullaby to the baby inside. It seemed good to end with the focus on the baby. We shared food together and I gave everyone a candle to light when I went into labour. We also decided who would telephone whom to spread the word when that happened.

I am sure that this preparation enabled me to approach the birth with more confidence and less fear. As the time drew near I felt more and more calm and deeply centred, and when I went into labour I was in a very positive frame of mind.

Including Older Siblings in the Preparations

When there are already children in the family, special care needs to be taken to make them feel part of the preparations to receive a new baby. Letting them come to midwives' appointments to hear the baby's heartbeat, and involving them in practical things like choosing toys or decorations for the baby's room are a good idea. Or you could take inspiration from Anita, who found a very visual way to express a welcome for her fourth child:

"We have a special table in our home, with displays that we change each season. Just the other day we cleared away the Easter things, and I thought it would be nice to make a welcome display for the new baby. For each of the children I've made a little felt baby in a walnut shell, so we set out the three babies in their shells, and added the new one. We found a stone egg, hung up a star and put a candle in a holder made of rose quartz. We'll have the candle lit during the birth."

* * *

During the last weeks of pregnancy, preparations on all levels become more intense and a woman can begin to enter an altered state, withdrawing from the normal tasks of the world, and attuning to the callings of her body and the child within. Thus we enter the world of the next chapter: birth.

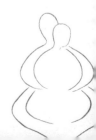

Chapter 7

Birth

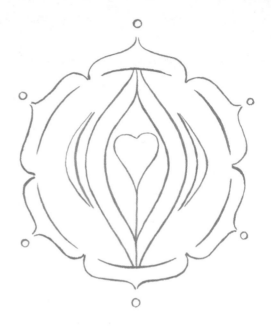

"There came to me assistance,
Mary fair and Bride;
As Anna bore Mary,
As Mary bore Christ,
As Eile bore John the Baptist
Without flaw in him,
Aid you me in my unbearing,
Aid me, O Bride"
        Gaelic Prayer, translated by A Carmichael[14]

Birth is the archetypal rite of passage for a woman, containing the essential elements of any ritual: separation from normal life, a profound transition during which the participants occupy a timeless time, followed by re-entry into society in a changed state. It can also be seen as a holy sacrament; the entry of a soul from another plane into this earthly dimension. Birth has always been, and still is, a momentous event, attended by great hopes as well as genuine risks, and one in which people call on a variety of powers for support and protection.

For the pre-Christian Celts in the Western Isles of Scotland, from whom the above prayer comes, it was the goddess Bride (or Brigid) who was known as the guardian of fertility. So powerful was her influence that when Christianity came to these people, a place was found for Bride at the centre of the nativity story, as midwife to Mary. When a woman was giving birth in a croft, the local 'knee-woman' (midwife) would go to the door with her arms open and call upon Bride to be present, and give her assistance. In this way, every birth, however humble, could partake of the divine.

Such a calling in of the spirit is still possible today, whether the birth is at home in a candle-lit pool, or by Caesarean in a brightly lit hospital. As it happens, I have experienced both of these kinds of birth, and can affirm that while one was definitely more beautiful than the other, they were equally remarkable and profound.

This chapter explores birth as a sacred time, set apart from the ordinary diurnal round, in which all the demands and challenges are held to be meaningful, and the birth itself is celebrated as miraculous. It will look at preparations for labour and take a glimpse into that strange land where women go during labour itself. It will pay some attention to the welcoming of the child in the first few minutes after birth. And then, because this exalted and topsy-turvy time extends far beyond the actual hours of birthing, it will consider the first few weeks with the new baby, and ways in which the new family can make conscious their re-entry into society.

Preparations

Preparations for birth interweave physical, mental, emotional, spiritual and practical matters.

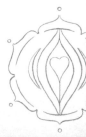

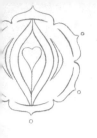

On the physical front, if you hope to give birth naturally, there are a wide variety of classes available to give your body the best chance of being fit and ready for labour. Many women find active birth, aquanatal or antenatal yoga classes help them to stay fit and flexible and provide some ideas for birthing positions. A class also introduces you to other mothers and mothers-to-be, and this network of people going through the same things as you may prove to be just as important as what is taught by the teachers.

There are important decisions to be made to set the mind at rest, such as where to have the baby, what kind of pain relief you want to be accessible, and who you want to be present at the birth. Your midwife may recommend writing these into a Birth Plan, which will be read by your team and should be honoured even if you are incapacitated and unable to make decisions at the time. If you wish your partner to be there, it's worth thinking about what support they might need, so that they can really be present for you when the time comes. If you plan to labour at home, you will need someone to hold the space for you, keeping a safe, quiet, undisturbed environment. You might decide to invite someone to be a birthing partner, either a reliable friend or a trusted professional. Because I wanted to have my first child at home, and was over thirty-five, I felt I needed a bit of extra support, so I hired a doula. The work of doulas, as described in the previous chapter, is to complement midwives by offering holistic practical and emotional support to women during pregnancy and birth. It was good to build a relationship with my doula in the months before the birth, through regular massages, and I found it comforting to know that, while I had no idea which midwives would attend my birth, she would definitely be there when the time came.

If I had to go into hospital, she would come with me. Some people go a step further and hire an independent midwife. This again is someone who will definitely be there for you, and who has a full medical training as well. A friend of mine, who had experienced a difficult first labour culminating in an emergency caesarean, opted to hire an independent midwife to deliver her second child. With this completely different outlook and strong support, she gave birth in a pool at home, with no complications.

Then there are emotional tugs and whispers that need to be attended to. All kinds of anxieties can impede a woman in labour, so it pays to give some time to addressing these in advance. Some women find hypnotherapy works well, and others use creative means like painting or modelling both their feared and ideal birth scenarios.[15]

Whatever kind of birth you are approaching, one thing you can do in preparation is make a mental rehearsal of it going well. This can be very reassuring, and particularly valid if your last birth experience was not so positive. You can combine this exercise with communicating with your baby about what to expect.

Visualisation for a Positive Birth Experience

Sitting or lying comfortably, begin by imagining the environment you hope to give birth in, and think of yourself there, feeling strong and believing in your power to give birth (or calm and trusting about undergoing an operation.)

Then begin to speak to the child, all the while visualising the birth going well and smoothly. I like speaking aloud, because it

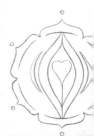

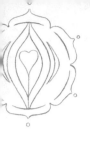

keeps me from drifting off mentally. Some people prefer to write things down, and others do better with pictures rather than words, so let yourself play and find your own way. Here is just one idea of what one might say:

"Hello little one, how are you doing? I hope you're happy there. It's nearly time for you to come out and meet us all. I think it's coming soon. I've got everything ready for you. You're going to make a big journey down a tunnel. There will be a lot of squeezing, but don't worry, you'll be fine. You're going to come out into the world! Your head will come out and I'll be able to feel it, and then all your body, and then you can come and lie with me and hear my voice. It might be a bit bright, and a bit surprising. It will be new and different, but we are so looking forward to seeing you and finding out who you are. Whenever you feel ready, my love, some day soon."

If your baby is overdue, you could also try checking in to see if there is anything holding her back from birth.

Preparations for a Home Birth

If you plan a home birth, the preparation of a place that is clean and safe for labouring is a necessary task. It also presents an opportunity to create a haven of beauty and inspiration, your own sacred space.

Lyn needed to construct a water pool in her newly rented house a few days before the baby was due, and turned the occasion into something of a housewarming party. The pool was filled, and children got in and splashed around, which filled the place with positive associations. When the time came to give birth, she had been burning frankincense for two days, and was, in her words, "really deep." She experienced being in the pool as like being in her mother's arms.

As the time for my first baby's birth came closer, I felt that I was beginning to retreat from the world a little more each day. A week before her due date I invited a friend to come and meditate with me in the room where she was going to be born. My partner Phil joined us, and we visualised a protective veil surrounding the house (which is a terrace on a busy street), imagining the room filling with love, calmness and light. I fixed a net curtain to the front window, despite having never wanted one before. Another couple I know hung silk scarves in the windows of their bedroom, thereby creating an inner sanctum for the first days with their son.

The following Sunday I had a 'show'. We meditated in the room again, this time using the Sufi chant 'Ya Fatah', which translates as 'The Opening of the Way'. It was during this meditation that it occurred to me I hadn't done one important bit of clearing, which was to empty my diary of commitments. I still had a recording session booked in for the following Tuesday. I rang and cancelled it, and felt that now the way was at last open. My last nesting obsession that day was to scrub the toilet bowl until it gleamed. This turned out to be a great idea, because that night my labour began and I spent a good deal of the next morning with my head down the loo.

If you lack the appropriate space for a home birth in your own house, it is possible to create a perfect birthing environment elsewhere. Sian lived in an upstairs flat but wanted to have a home birth with a birthing pool. Since a birthing pool is heavy and needs

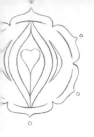

to be situated in a downstairs room, Sian arranged to use a spare bedroom in a friend's house.

"I wanted to make the room cosy – a creative, safe place for me. I chose red, orange and yellow fabrics to warm up the room. Mum helped me decorate it with daffodils and pussy willow from her garden, so there was something of outside inside, rooting me to things I felt close to. It felt very protective, like being within a womb myself. The room was lit by candlelight, and it was very beautiful. It was a place I felt happy to be naked in; a place I'd have been happy to make love in. Doing this was claiming the event as sacred – pregnancy isn't an illness, and birth doesn't have to happen in a sterile environment."

Anita was due her third child in high summer, and didn't feel comfortable about being in the house.

"I asked the midwife how she would feel if I had the baby in the garden, and she was alright about it. That August it poured with rain, but we made a lovely shelter, and I had the baby there. While I was pregnant I collected birch leaves from a branch blown off in a storm. Birches are seen as symbols of new life, because the birch is the first tree to colonise an area of scrubland that is returning to forest. I pressed them, and on the morning that my daughter was born, my two sons brought the leaves out of the flower press and scattered them around us."

Even if you are planning a home birth, it may set your mind at rest to have visited your local hospital so that it's not a completely foreign experience if you find it necessary to transfer there during labour. Likewise, there is no harm in finding out about Caesarean Section, just in case.

Preparations for a Hospital Birth

If you choose to give birth in hospital, it is worth seeing if you can visit the delivery suite in advance to have a look at the environment, meet some of the staff and ask any questions you might have about how things are done. The more information and understanding you have, the more empowered you will be to ask for what you need. For example, you may be able to request dimmed lighting, and in some places you can play your own music. There is nothing to stop you bringing in some flowers, a picture, or photograph if those things help you to claim the space and make you more comfortable, and you can usually wear your own clothes, even if they offer you a hospital gown. Do ask about moving around during labour too, and check that any beanbags or birthing balls provided are actually firm enough to be useful. If possible, try to talk to other people who have given birth in that setting and ask what they suggest you bring in. Extra pillows, and some high quality snacks and fresh juice drinks are often recommended, as are essential oils of rose and jasmine to inhale from a cotton handkerchief. (Sometimes midwives can supply these oils, if asked in advance.)

Preparations for a Caesarean Birth

Some people find themselves going through an emergency Caesarean with no warning at all, but if the operation is planned, you have an opportunity to prepare yourself and the baby. A Caesarean presents different challenges to a woman than those of a natural birth, but it is still a profound surrender, as I discovered when fate decreed my second child would be delivered this way.

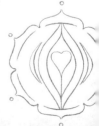

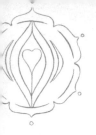

Well into the second term of my pregnancy, I was found to have placenta previa; a condition where the placenta covers the cervix and physically prevents the baby being born through the birth canal. In times gone by, this was a very serious condition, usually resulting in the death of the baby (and sometimes the mother too from haemorrhage). I had no choice but to put my faith in the medics, who scheduled a Caesarean at thirty-eight weeks and kept me in hospital for five weeks in the run up to it, in case of sudden bleeding. For someone who likes being in control, that was not an easy task. I found it much more comfortable to trust the flow of my body to take me through labour, than to trust the anaesthetists, surgeons, nurses and drugs to take me safely through this operation. And yet, when the time came, I wanted to be willing. Just as in my preparation for a natural birth, I did not want to add resistance into the equation. Perhaps the surrender to a planned operation is harder because you are not in an altered state at the start of it. Thus the meditation I suggest here is to cultivate acceptance. If you take this up as a daily practice in the time before the birth it will be easier to apply in the more intense environment of the operating theatre.

Meditation before a Caesarean

There is no need to sit still to carry out this practice, as sitting can be very uncomfortable in late pregnancy. The meditation can be done while walking, lying, or standing at the bus stop – whenever you remember.

The practice is simply to nod the head, and say inwardly, 'Yes.' Whatever is going on, whether it be delightful, or thoroughly unpleasant, breathe into it and think, 'OK, this is what is happening now.' Pay attention to each sense in turn: what can you see? Hear? Smell? Taste? Feel? Notice your thoughts, and remember that they are not you, they are just thoughts. It becomes quite a liberation not to hold on to your judgements about things, but to witness instead how sensations arise and then pass away.

When you find yourself feeling anxious about the coming operation, just remind yourself to nod and say, 'Yes.' When you are putting on the ridiculous surgical stockings, think, 'Yes,' and allow yourself to smile. When the epidural needle is going in, breathe deeply and think 'Yes, this pain is like a contraction and will pass.' When you are numb from the chest down, being lifted onto the trolley and wheeled into the operating theatre, just think, 'yes, yes, yes.'

Because I had made a birthing necklace in advance of the my first baby's birth (see Mother Blessings in the previous chapter) I brought this into the hospital and hung it on my wall. Even though I couldn't wear it during the operation, it helped me to remember that this would still be a birth; a challenging and yet joyous event, and one for which the qualities of love, going with the flow, majesty and a sense of humour would be just as important as during a natural labour.

A few days before my planned Caesarean I had a visit in hospital from a friend, Tess Ward, who is also the hospital chaplain. Tess is a rare human being who works within the church but maintains an appreciation of the divine feminine. She asked if she could give a blessing to me and the baby before birth, and I readily agreed. I was by that time so accustomed to the hands of midwives hooking me up to ultrasound scans, and checking my blood pressure and temperature, that it was a relief to feel a hand on my belly that spoke

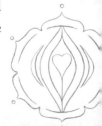

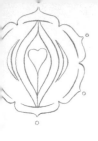

of love and wonder and beauty, rather than the functionality of the body. Tess rubbed my forehead and belly with scented oil and laid flowers from her garden on my bump. We shut our eyes and she asked Mother Spirit to surround the baby and me, to keep us safe through the operation, to bring blessing on the hands of the surgeon and the skill of the midwives. This brought me peace in the hours leading up to the operation, and helped me to face it with quiet confidence, feeling protected.

In the event, everything went smoothly, and in a very short space of time my blood-and-vermix-smeared little girl lay against my chest, like some subterranean animal shutting her eyes against the brightness.

If, like me, you are a nature-lover who finds beauty in the natural order of things, it may be hard to accept that a medicalised birth can be as valid. Yet who are we to limit the scope of what we call Nature, or indeed Spirit? One woman told me how, amidst the rush of her emergency C-section, she saw each doctor with their angelic counterpart. For her, the operating theatre was a temple of light and song, filled with beings of light.

Labour

As the baby's due date nears there is a natural turning in of the mother's energy. I have seen this in many women, who become less and less of this world, more dreamy and withdrawn, and move towards an altered state as their due date approaches. It's important to rest as much as possible at this time, to conserve energy for labour. There is also a gathering excitement as the moment approaches. The last piece of advice my favourite midwife gave me the day before Heather's due date, was simply, 'stay in touch with yourself, and stay in touch with the baby'. The evening before labour started I was sitting quietly, and I felt either some part of me or the baby say, 'I'm ready'. I wasn't surprised to wake a few hours later with deep lower back pain heralding the first contractions. As it was night-time and the contractions were not strong, I stayed in bed drifting in and out of sleep and dream. At one point I felt as if the whole of me was a great uterus contracting.

By early morning, the contractions were too strong to stay in bed. It was a beautiful June morning so I went into the garden and found myself happily pulling bindweed out from around a peony rose that I'd planted in my mother's honour. I sang songs and felt close to her. As contractions strengthened I started to feel less and less rational. I kept thinking I might make bread, but actually I just moved from one room to another not really knowing what I was doing, picking things up, putting them down, feeling sick, being sick, thinking about making bread again, never even getting the flour out of the cupboard. For a short time I was on the edge of feeling frightened, fearing that if someone saw me they would think I was going out of my mind. Fortunately, my partner, doula and midwife all seemed quite unperturbed by my unusual behaviour, so I was able to relax into it. Some enlightened midwives see this as their ideal role: if labour is progressing well, they are there to hold a safe space for the woman while she lets go of her rational mind and accesses the more primal part of the brain-body, which knows how to birth, in her own unique style. I wonder whether this is one of the aspects of birth that a modern hospital system, which has

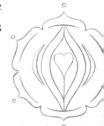

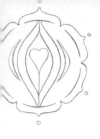

to function according to timetables and regulations, finds hardest to support. Furthermore, there are not many opportunities in our mainstream culture for people to experience this liminal state, so it may be viewed with suspicion. Perhaps the only people who might recognise it as a 'high' state, which one can visit and return from, are artists, manic-depressives and people who take recreational psychedelics.

It should be no surprise to find, then, a volume of extraordinary birth stories and a revolutionary spiritual approach to midwifery coming out of 1970s California. In her book, *Spiritual Midwifery*, Ina May Gaskin tells the story of three hundred God-fearing hippies who lived and travelled in a caravan of 50 converted school buses.[16] Families among them fell pregnant, and, as with the rest of their unconventional lifestyle, they took things into their own hands, and delivered the babies on the buses themselves, through a mixture of faith in nature and God. They coined the word 'rushes' to describe what we normally call contractions, and many of the women talk about it being 'Holy' or 'psychedelic' and about becoming 'telepathic' with all the people in the room.

That level of ecstasy wasn't quite my experience, but I did continue to inhabit a somewhat altered state as my labour continued, with me getting into the delicious warm birthing pool in my candle-lit living room, and I began to move my hips in the water, dancing with the sensations of gentle contractions. I listened to whale and dolphin voices on a CD, and felt these wild and intelligent creatures calling me to a deep knowing part of myself. Phil got into the pool too and held me, giving affectionate kisses in between contractions. As things intensified, I asked for violin music, and felt the exquisite beauty of Beethoven and Brahms' violin concertos as never before, full of the pain and bliss of life itself. Time passed, the contractions strengthened, Phil found a way to push hard against my lower back, which helped with the pain.

More than anything, what I needed to labour was an unbroken focus and no distractions. The moments I found hardest were when anyone took me back into time. I didn't want to know how long I had been going, or how long they thought I had to go, and I didn't want to know how dilated I was. Within time, I was my normal self again and my normal self couldn't cope. Luckily my midwives were very respectful of my wishes, and took a very quiet role, just observing, taking notes and being there in case of need. I hardly noticed when they changed shift. I didn't want any music at this point. I got through the contractions by counting aloud – I hadn't planned to do this, but it seemed to help me to know that they would peak and pass after sixteen counts. Later, I could only count to five and go back to the beginning, keeping my sights on a nearer goal. After a good while of strong contractions, I reached a surprisingly comfortable plateau, where I actually dosed off a little, then perked up and asked for a cup of tea, and some different music.

There was a moment when I felt stuck, and didn't know what to do any more. Having asked for everyone in the room to keep a respectful distance, I suddenly felt furious that there were at least four people in the room, none of whom seemed to be helping at all! I think this is probably what is called transition, and for me it was the hardest part. My lesson at that point was to quit doing it on my own and ask for help. Coming to the rescue, my doula then made her one major intervention, which was to twist a towel firmly, give me one

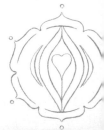

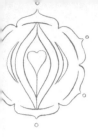

end to pull, while squatting, as she pulled the other end. Somehow that seemed to show my body how to push. Suddenly certain that the baby was a girl, I started talking to her and encouraging her out, "Come on girl, come on, we can do this" and interspersed with this I found myself chanting the Sufi words 'Ya Hai', which means 'Life' or 'The Divine Life'. It's a very strong sound, a bit like the noise a martial arts expert makes when he slices planks with his bare hand, and it felt really good to use it at that point. I did indeed feel that I was partaking of divine life at that moment. It was much more active and less a surrender than the part before.

Perhaps I could have used a little more hands-on help at that point, because suddenly I could feel the baby's head, but I didn't manage to communicate that. After a few more big pushes (which did hurt, I have to say!) out she came, a little askew and tearing me considerably. Phil caught her and raised her above the water, where she made a triumphant shout. After that she was very alert and did not cry at all. She fixed us with a bright and intelligent gaze and then tried latching on to Phil's nipple, while I became involved in a bizarre game of Twister, trying to follow the midwife's instructions to climb over the umbilical cord so that we could all sit together.

Labour tests a woman's resources to the limit, and how she responds to it is so personal, I cannot prescribe anything or make any suggestions as to how to do it. What I do believe, though, is that given the right environment you will find your way. Even without it, you may reach beyond yourself. A woman told me of her experience in a hospital ward at night waiting to go down to the delivery suite. Midwives examined her and told her she had a long time to wait, and wasn't dilating at all, so she stayed put by herself, but was having strong contractions. Whenever they came on she went into a dream of running on a beach. By the time she was taken down to the delivery suite she was just about ready to give birth, and had done all that labour on her own. Another woman in early stages of labour in bed alone talked of seeing wheels turning, fire and darkness. When she breathed it was like opening a window. She realised afterwards that sensation was her cervix opening.

We know that dilation and contraction of the cervix is affected by the mother's moods. Labour can slow down or stop altogether if a mother feels threatened or disturbed from her concentration. In *Spiritual Midwifery*, midwife Ina May Gaskin tells the story of a mother whose labour, which had been progressing well, seemed to get stuck; the cervix was fully dilated but the baby wasn't moving down the birth canal.[17] Rather than move into a medical intervention, Ina May noticed how the woman's face seemed pinched around her mouth. On an impulse she asked if she had ever told her husband that she loved him. It turned out that she hadn't. After a few moments, the words came, her face softened, and a powerful contraction began to push her baby out.

This illustrates how complex the factors are that affect the progress of a birth. Birth is a truly holistic event, in which the boundaries between mind and body, within and without, spiritual and material seem to dissolve away. It makes a lot of difference whether one frames the pain of a contraction as an intense experience, which will pass in time, or a terrible affliction, which one might not survive. It is the difference between saying "Good contraction, excellent" rather than "Oh it looks like you're having a lot of trouble there, would you like some pain relief?"

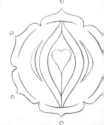

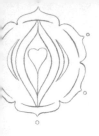

As an inspiring contrast from another culture, we could look at the traditional belly dance of pre-Islamic Arab communities. Women and girls would be taught the complex moves including hip circles and belly rolls in advance of becoming pregnant, as a way to tone the muscles and teach the body the way of bringing a baby out. When a woman laboured, all the women would gather in concentric circles around her to do the dance and encourage her. Their presence was a strong reminder of the woman's place within the shared circle of women's experience. The dance itself, in addition to being a physical workout, was a celebration of maternity, and of the shared suffering and joy that attends the birth of a new soul.

When there is a strong team around a labouring woman, they can somehow share the labour, even to the point of feeling some of the pain. Fathers sometimes genuinely feel sympathetic pangs when their partners are labouring, and birthing partners and other birth attendants sometimes also take on some of the pain and appear to carry it for the woman giving birth.

Sian, who gave birth in the pool, said: "I felt so animal. I'd kept my sounds really low, keeping it calm, riding it. There was a moment with everyone around the pool, supporting me, but the sensation was inside me, I couldn't get away from it. The naturalness of it – it strips away all civilizedness and leaves you connected to your animal power. Fundamentally it was not a passive thing to be suffered but an act of creativity. I felt so vindicated. I was euphoric, and I've been on a high ever since. I remember climbing a mountain in the Himalayas and thinking, that's the hardest thing apart from giving birth. If you've done that, you can do anything."

The Child's Arrival and the First Weeks

How a child is treated in the first moments of his or her life says a good deal about the culture he or she is born into. In a modern hospital the baby is often cleaned, weighed, tested for vital signs, given a score out of five, and then injected with vitamin K before even feeling the hands of his mother. It is possible to express your preferences about this in a birth plan. If you have a home birth there is a lot more scope for a gentler beginning, with lowered lights and skin-to-skin contact straight away, but even in hospital these moments immediately after labour can be a precious time, as Zara describes here:

"When Rowan arrived, we held him flesh to flesh and sang to him. He would have known those songs from the womb because all through the pregnancy I had sung songs, with names for both a boy and a girl. My husband said I sang him into the world. It wasn't conscious, but I suppose those songs express our worldview, so it was probably the beginning of teaching him what we believe in. It was also a kind of thanksgiving to the universe that he was safe and well."

There are some interesting customs that show how a worldview may be shared with the child in its first instants. Many Muslims believe that Allah should be the first word heard by a newborn, so the call to prayer is spoken into the right ear of the baby at birth, and the command to rise and worship is spoken into its left ear. A Hindu child may have the sacred word 'OM' written on its tongue with honey or ghee.[18] For others, the child is the one showing the way to the divine. As Toby said of his first child, "He was the guru, fresh from God, from the 'Isness'."

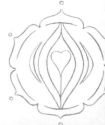

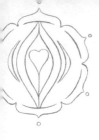

The first hours and days after the birth of a new child are intense for everyone closely involved, especially when it is a first child in the family. People have all kinds of experiences, but perhaps my own emotional journey after my first child is not that unusual. After Heather's peaceful birth at home, I had to transfer to hospital to have stitches, and then, because I had lost a lot of blood and felt very weak, I opted to recover for a couple of days in a local community hospital. During this time and the following weeks at home I felt every bit as challenged as I had done in labour. I've always found it easier to pull the stops out for a big occasion than to deal with day-to-day life. To begin with, I was elated by the birth, bewitched by my daughter and in love with my partner as the hormones swam around my bloodstream. On about day three I wept nearly all day, missing my mother. When we came home I was anxious beyond reason about almost everything, which made it hard to sleep even though I was exhausted. It was hard to switch off when I knew I would be woken again at any moment by a demanding babe. Breastfeeding was hard, and everything hurt. Then I developed an infection and lost any ground I had gained in terms of strength and energy. I couldn't imagine ever riding a bicycle or making love again. I didn't know if I would ever feel normal. In truth I think you don't ever return to your body as it was before the pregnancy. Once that threshold is passed, you are in a new and unfamiliar land. You do recover, but you are remade in a different form.

Lyn: "When you've become a mother, every single cell in your body and your soul is different. It's like you've been turned inside out. How you look at the world changes. I had to come to terms with being a woman. I'd always been a bit of a tomboy, and I was suddenly exposed as a woman. The old mask didn't work any more – everything had to be absolutely real. I learned what fear is, what insecurity is. I didn't have the energy to wear a mask. It brought me down into real life with a bump."

During this time I found the lessons of my birthing necklace kept coming back to me: 'Go with the flow', 'surrender', 'don't try to be perfect', 'keep a sense of humour'. Whenever I did these things I found that everything was actually fine. The flow of people arriving to help at opportune moments, with a dish of food here, or some well-chosen words there, was truly extraordinary. What I found so hard to do was to relax into being looked after and trust everyone to manage, while I healed. This was probably the biggest lesson I had to learn during these high times. A dear friend came and held my head and listened while I complained that I didn't know what I was doing, that I was scared by everything feeling out of my control. She christened this a state of 'Divine Flailing'. Somehow that made it easier to bear.

After a Traumatic Birth

The natural flow of birth can be interrupted in all kinds of ways, and when this happens the mother may feel cheated, angry and upset, especially if she has cherished an ideal of a particular kind of birth. If she is in physical pain as well, it can be particularly difficult, and it may take a long time to come to terms with what has happened. In such a situation a ritual can play a role in helping recovery, by offering a way of taking control again, and redressing the balance after a traumatic delivery.

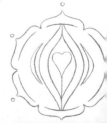

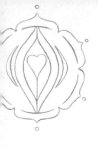

Ruth: "Ben's birth was quite violent. The midwife insisted that there should be electrodes on the baby's head, and that meant that I couldn't move naturally. I lost control of the pain, and ended up asking for an epidural. In the end it was a forceps delivery, and I was almost yanked onto the floor when he was pulled out. Ben's head was cut, and I also had to have stitches. I was in quite a strange state for some days afterwards. I was overjoyed but strangely anxious. Everything slowed down and I was acutely aware of every sensation.

When Ben was about a week old I did a little ceremony for him. I decorated his chair with flowers, placed all the congratulations cards around him, lit candles and burned incense. For the first time since the birth I got out of my T-shirt and dressed myself in special clothes, even though I was on my own. I made sandwiches and brought honey to symbolise nourishment, and a glass of Ouzo, brought back from a recent holiday, to celebrate. I sang a few songs and said a few words. When my partner came home he joined in. It was a little holiday from the demanding round-the-clock feeding and looking after the baby. I wanted to mark Ben's arrival, and to put the trauma of the birth behind us. The flowers symbolised fertility and my desire to be in harmony with nature. I knew we wouldn't have a religious ceremony for him, and we were not in the habit of having parties, so this was my way of welcoming him."

After a Caesarean

However well-prepared one is, and however good the obstetric team, a Caesarean is still a major operation and giving the body some opportunity to release fears afterwards is important. This happened for me in quite a strange and spontaneous way. When the nurse took off the dressing from my wound, I went into an uncontrollable shaking and shivering fit, which lasted about ten minutes. That night, still in hospital with my new baby, I dreamt of having sex with two nurses and woke, at the point of orgasm, shaking violently again, and quite frightened! Reflecting on this with a friend afterwards we wondered if my body, denied its experience of ecstatic labour, had provided me with a dream that allowed me to feel some of those intense sensations. Like any woman after a Caesarean, I was sore, bruised and numb in the abdomen for many weeks. It takes time to recover strength and confidence in that part of the body, and longer to feel whole and sexy again. I found a gentle hand resting on my womb helped me to cry and release difficult feelings, and Reiki from a friend was very helpful. Although you can carry on with your life pretty well after about six weeks, I think it takes about a year to fully mend. It's very hard to take time out for yourself when you are looking after a young baby, but if you possibly can, your body will be grateful.

Confinement

There is a great deal of variation in different cultures around the world as to when women return to their normal activities. Some women are not allowed the luxury of time off to recover, and are expected to be back at their work in the fields within days. But in very many places a period of separation from work and normal society is preserved by strong tradition or taboo. For example, Roma women with newborn children are isolated from the community and not

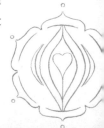

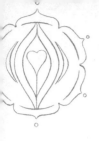

allowed to touch kitchen utensils for four to six weeks, until after the child's baptism. After this time, the woman washes herself in the river and everything she has used since giving birth is burnt or thrown away.[19]

In much of Asia, a tradition of one month's confinement is still followed, although with a good deal of modern variations in strictness. In its traditional form the woman is not allowed to leave the house, bathe or wash her hair, do any exercise, read books or watch TV. She must eat only certain foods, which are considered warming, and drink nothing but a warm tea made from red dates. Friends and relatives come, bringing gifts for mother and child. The mother can achieve this degree of rest because she is attended by another woman, called a 'Pui Yuet'; either a professional paid for the job, or member of the family, who cooks and looks after the baby. The purpose of this confinement is to bring the mother's body back into balance after the exertions of pregnancy and labour, specifically to keep her warm and to drive out 'Fong', the element of wind in Chinese traditional medicine. Women who do not follow the rules are deemed to be at risk from rheumatism, headaches and backache in much later life and many young women consider that a month of inconvenience and discomfort is a price worth paying to keep them healthy in older age.

Although in rather an extreme form, these customs speak of the need for the new mother and baby to be kept separate from the rest of the world for a while. In modern life we have to be careful not to get busy too quickly, even with visitors and well wishers, who, no matter how kind, can be exhausting.

Burying the Placenta

One ritual I did in the first week of Heather's life was to bury her placenta in the garden. We had kept it in the fridge with a view to frying up a little bit for me to replenish lost nutrients. Whilst that might have been a good idea, by the time I returned from the community hospital, it was a few days old and I wasn't sure I fancied it any more! So Phil cleared a space in the garden by removing a shrub that had seen better days, and dug a hole ready for the placenta together with a small fig tree, which had been in a pot ready to be planted out as soon as we could think of a place to put it. We were going to do this on our own, but it happened that a Jewish friend dropped by at exactly that moment, so she became a natural part of our little ceremony. She helped me to find a half-remembered passage from the Old Testament Song of Songs, which expressed my rapturous love for our newborn, whose young voice in contented sleep seemed to me like the cooing of a dove, and which also speaks of fig tree putting forth its leaves (Song of Songs Chapter 2 Verses 10-14). Then we each spoke spontaneously about our wishes for Heather, based around earth (that she might be nourished by earth and enjoy the fruits of the soil all her life), water (that she might not go thirsty, that she might have fun playing with water), fire (that she might be blessed with warmth, passion and creativity) and air (that she may breathe clean air and know freedom). Putting the placenta in the earth felt a good landmark for me, demonstrating how she was now going to be nourished more directly by the earth, and other elements, rather than via me. It also made a strong link between her and our home, enacting an exchange of energy with the place that sustains and shelters us. In the two years since then she has certainly

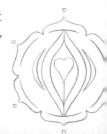

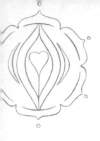

enjoyed many fruits from the garden, including an apple from our tree, which was her first taste of food other than milk.

I was grateful for the advice of a friend who had organised a bigger welcoming ceremony for their first child a few weeks after the birth, which included a placenta burial. She felt that it was too soon to be so public, and also that the placenta was too raw and personal to be widely seen. Having done it myself, I am sure this is right: if you want to do a ritual involving the placenta, it needs to be quite a private event. (Of course, you can freeze the placenta if you want to wait a little longer before dealing with it, but be careful that it doesn't become a long-forgotten biohazard at the bottom of your freezer!)

Re-entry into Society

After a period of lying low and quietly getting used to life with a new baby, there comes a time to step back into wider society. For us, this usually goes by without ceremony, but there are many precedents for this occasion being marked, as an opportunity for thanksgiving or celebration.

In rural Uganda, when a mother who has recently given birth leaves the hut for the first time, she wears special clothes, and has earned the right to carry a ceremonial staff. She is welcomed back into the community at the market place, where songs are sung to her, celebrating her courage and achievement. The songs are just like those sung to warriors returning from battle, and reflect the fact that women in childbirth braved death, just as much as men in battle did.[20]

In Jewish and Christian traditions, the emphasis was rather different, with a woman deemed as 'unclean' for a set period (40 days if the child was a boy, 80 if it was a girl) after the birth, until she made offerings at the temple to free her from 'pollution'. Nowadays a new Jewish mother may go to the 'Mikvah' for a ritual bath, instead of making an offering. In medieval Christianity there was a service with the unwieldy title of: 'The Thanksgiving of Women After Child Birth, Commonly Called the Churching Of Women'. This was carried out 40 days after birth, and was the first time the woman was allowed into church to receive Holy Communion. There was no direct reference to ritual cleansing; rather it was a thanksgiving to God for delivering the woman from 'the great paine and peryl of childe birth', and was performed even if the child had not survived.[21] Whilst the liturgy for this service has been included in recent prayer books, it has fallen out of usage in the West. In the East it continues, and since the church is a centre for social as well as religious life, the occasion is an opportunity for meeting up with friends and family and for lavish feasting.

Modern women may not face the prospect of death through childbirth so starkly, but its shadow is still there, and there is still a part of us that needs to be honoured and acknowledged for surviving the ordeal of the birth. A gift from a partner gives reassurance that he will be there for this new stage of the relationship, loving the mother as he loved the maiden. Gifts from the new mother's own mother, or mother-in-law, demonstrate the new status that the woman has attained in the family.

About six weeks after Heather was born we decided to throw a little party in our garden. Up until then we had been very reclusive,

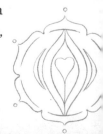

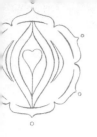

and even had a notice on the door asking people not to call in without making an arrangement first. It was a very simple affair, with tea and cake for a few friends, but it was our 'coming out' party, and a chance to thank people for the support they'd offered in the first weeks. I find it interesting that we set the date for this event at about 40 days after Heather's birth, without being conscious of the traditions above. Perhaps there is some kind of natural shift at that point, which the ancient traditions honoured.

Sharing Birth Stories

All birth stories are powerful: not the dispassionate obstetric notes that state the time, degrees of dilation and progress of labour, but the stories of the mother's inner experience, of the mental places she went to during contractions, the things that distracted her, the moments of wonder, the things that made her angry, the surprises. These stories are ours to share if we choose to. For an expectant first-time mother, positive birth stories are part of a diet that nourishes a perception of women as capable birth-givers, and helps her to imagine herself in that role.

They could be shared verbally as part of a mother blessing ceremony, or they could be written down in a book that's passed from mother to mother among friends. The birthing pool I used to give birth to my first child has a list of names of the children born in it on the side. There is a book to accompany the pool too, for the mothers to write down their stories. Of course it is hard to find the time to do this – many pages of the book are still blank. But we try.

I have also heard of a necklace being passed on in a similar way. A woman wears the necklace during labour, and when the child is born she gains the right to add a bead. The string of beads comes to stand for all the children born into the tribe, and is offered to each woman as a mark of her belonging to a community of mothers.

* * *

The experience of birth is on the one hand universal, but on the other hand completely unique to each woman and each baby. It is the most wonderfully unpredictable event, and even to scratch the surface of the different cultural traditions surrounding it shows how it is interpreted in a multitude of different ways. The western woman living in early twenty-first century is lucky to be able to exercise a good deal of choice about her options for giving birth.

Even so, birth is a challenge, as is motherhood. The lessons of the first are sharp and fast, while those of the other are spread out over days and years and require a different kind of stamina. We can approach birth as an inconvenience and an ordeal standing between us and the prize of a child, but to do so robs birth of its power to teach us what we need to know to become mothers. If instead we submit to its mysteries and surrender to its sufferings, we invite initiation to a deeper understanding and acceptance of life. My sense is that if we set out to do this consciously, we attract choruses of angels who make the path clear for us and sing us on our way.

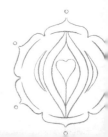

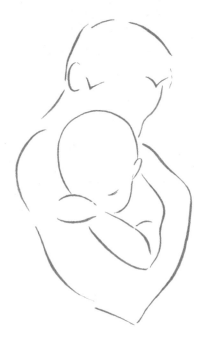

Chapter 8

Becoming
a Father

"Becoming a father isn't difficult,
But it's very difficult to become a father."
Wilhelm Busch, 1877

Becoming a father is not the fundamental journey of transformation that a woman makes to become a mother, but it is nevertheless a profound transition that merits both reflection and celebration. Before and after birth, when attention is naturally focussed on the mother, the father's needs may become sidelined. Yet, if we are to encourage men to become engaged and supportive fathers, they too need to be affirmed as they make this important step.

The stories in this chapter are of men who are consciously exploring what it means to become a father. In most cases they did not learn this from their own fathers, who too often were distant or absent altogether from their lives as children. In any case, there has been so much change in the roles available to women in recent years that men have been forced to reassess their role in raising children too. In the days of a crisis of identity for men, and in a context where a great number of children are sadly growing up without a steady father figure in their lives, these men are the trailblazers.

Before Conception

The conscious acceptance of fathering begins with a serious contemplation before embarking on the journey. For some this is part of the decision to get married.

Martin: "It took three years to make our wedding ceremony come about, but through the making of that ritual I was changed on a cellular level. In my centre, I decided to stay with this woman, and all that comes with that. As soon as we were married we stopped using contraceptives."

For others it directs the course of their relationships.

Thomas: "When I was in my mid 30s I thought for a long time about whether I wanted to have children. I asked all the parents I knew whether they would recommend it. They all said that it had completely changed their lives, that it was far more difficult than they had imagined, but that they would not have chosen otherwise. I went on retreat and spent two weeks meditating with this question. When I thought about becoming a father, I felt rage at the thought of another human being depriving me of my autonomy. Bizarrely, at the end of the two weeks I decided I did want to have children. I am a link in a chain that goes back millions of years, and I didn't want it to end here. Making that decision transformed the way I dealt with

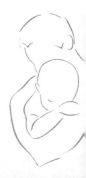

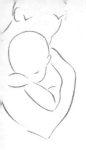

relationships. I ended the relationship I was in because my partner didn't want to have children. Shortly after that I met the woman who is now my wife and the mother of my son."

During Pregnancy

Many men now attend antenatal classes and doctor's appointments with their partner. Modern technology provides the possibility for a prospective father to perceive the unborn baby with his own senses much earlier than would be possible without its aid.

Martin: "For me the idea of the baby was abstract until I heard its heartbeat. Seven hours later I was suddenly struck by an overwhelming love, an unspeakable devotion to the source of that sound."

Others bond with the child in the womb by touch, or by voice.

Hugh: " We both chanted to the child, while he was in the womb, and again later when he was born. I went to see him in intensive care – he was in one of those strange sandwich box type incubators, and I thought, "What do you say, when you see your child for the first time?" So I chanted, and he opened his eyes. When he was older we would chant if he got distressed, and that seemed to calm him."

When I was pregnant with Heather, Phil and I sometimes lit a candle and sat together in silence with him behind me, supporting me.

Phil: "Doing this practice helped me realise what my role as a father was. I thought of it like an onion. In the centre of the onion is the baby who's directly supported by the mother. My role was to support the mother, and protect them both. As the pregnancy progressed I found my protectiveness intensified. Just walking down a footpath and seeing a gang of boisterous youths approaching could bring me almost to the point of violence!"

Preparing for Birth

In the knowledge that a serious change of lifestyle is approaching, some men feel the need to take some time out to prepare.

Luke: "Before I became a dad, I left the antenatal classes I had been attending with Catherine and went off for ten days on my own cycling around Southern France and the Pyrenees. It was very self-indulgent – a final solitary adventure before fatherhood. Catherine was very supportive of it. Funnily enough, six months later we went back with the baby Josh and two friends and cycled around the same area with him in a child seat. It was almost as if the pre-birth trip had been a recce for his first adventure, though I didn't know it at the time."

For some, it was important to spend time with other fathers. Jake decided to call a council of fathers and friends to support him in the preparation of becoming a father.

Jake: "When Rhiannon organised a baby shower with her women friends, she suggested I do something with the men, and I thought it was a good idea. I made a list of the people I wanted to be there. I thought first of the dads and step-dads who I knew, and felt connected to. I also invited some men who weren't dads, partly because I valued their thinking, and partly because I thought they would help to balance the group. There was a wide range of people from very different backgrounds, and I was worried they might not get on with each other, and that the conversation might stay at a superficial level. That's the hard bit about creating your own rite of

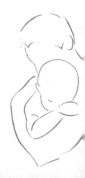

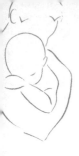

passage – you don't want to be pretentious, so you have to keep it light and casual, but at the same time it needs to be real.

We met in someone's house, and people brought food and drink with them. There was a lot of talking in the kitchen, then we gathered and sat in a big circle. There were 15 of us. I told them why they were there: that I was about to be a father and I wanted the benefit of their experience and wisdom. I just asked them to say something they found really good about being a dad and something they found hard, and to speak for roughly five minutes. I asked my best friend to speak first because I knew he would set a high tone. After that we pulled names out of a hat so that no one had to think about their turn coming up next.

As it happened, the first three men spoke about how great being a father is, how much they loved their children. Then the fourth man to speak was someone whose child had been killed in a car crash. He spoke very strongly, and he cried. That took it to another level of emotional honesty. One of the men who wasn't a father spoke about his relationship with his own dad. Another man spoke about the struggle he had to connect to his baby.

None of those men had ever been brought together and recognised as dads before. It was very powerful, being with other men, sharing feelings and being listened to. We were – and still are – trying to create a community of dads. Ideally your own dad would be there for you at this time, but when I ask my dad for advice, it's very superficial.

It made me feel very positive about becoming a father. I felt safe and confident in the support of other dads, and it was reassuring to hear that they had all been there and survived. They were telling me, when the time comes, you will have enough love. I knew they were telling me something that I wouldn't understand until I experienced it, and they were right.

When Anna came out and I held her against my chest, so fragile and needy, suddenly there was no mystery or problem – it was just obvious: I have to take care of this child. Obviously I'll rearrange my life. Obviously I'll put her first,"

Birth and Afterwards

Men who participate in the births of their children are frequently awed by the experience. Phil was very involved in the birth of our first daughter.

Phil: "Going to birth preparation classes helped me to understand what I could do during the birth. My job, when labour started, was to get the birthing pool ready, make a few phone calls, make the midwives welcome, and just be there. I was involved all the way through, from first being woken with the news that labour had started, through to getting into the birthing pool, holding Jackie while she relaxed between contractions, pressing acupressure points on her lower back during contractions until my thumbs ached, and finally catching Heather when she came out and cutting the cord.

The biggest surprise for me was how sensual it was being in the birthing pool together. There was closeness and physical contact and I felt very, very present. It was incredibly erotic. Being so intimate with Jackie at that time, seeing the expression on her face, the perspiration on her brow, an expression of her woman-

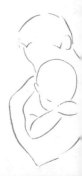

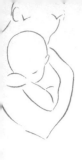

ness presented in that stark naked way, all of that helped me to understand the transition between not being a mother and being a mother. I wasn't detached from it and isolated, as I imagine someone would be who was kept waiting in a corridor."

Birth can also be a difficult time for a man, watching his partner labour and feeling powerless to protect her from pain. Added to which, with the arrival of the child, a man may need reassurance about his importance and recognition of his new role as father.

Hugh Dunford Wood is a painter from Shepherd's Bush who runs mentoring groups and visions quests for men and boys.

Hugh: " When I became a father, a very primitive urge arose to protect, provide for and shelter the family. It is a subservient role, to take care of the mother, who is taking care of the child, but that responsibility has a depth to it that you can't understand if you haven't had children. The difficulty is that a man feels he wants to be rewarded for taking on this role, but at this moment his partner's attention is elsewhere, monopolized by the baby. In addition, his relationship with the baby is less intimate than the mother's.

Just as a woman needs a doula (birthing partner), a man ideally wants a brother or mentor around at this time to tell him that he's doing well, and to tell him that this particular situation isn't going to last forever. He needs to be told that he will get his reward in ample terms later, as long as he can act with integrity now. Becoming a father is not a straight journey, it's more elliptical, and the blessings take time to emerge."

* * *

Children need fathers. Certainly, there are single mothers who make a fantastic job of raising children alone, and lesbian couples who create loving stable homes, but every child who grows up without a father figure experiences some kind of loss. Perhaps the saddest loss is when a father who is in the picture is distant or inaccessible to his children, for this is the man's loss as well as the child's.

Wherever men are finding ways to support each other to become more engaged fathers, through men's groups, rituals or informal networks, they, their partners and their children all benefit. As a woman, I rejoice to see men deliberately and proudly becoming fathers and stepfathers; their work is a gift to our future generations.

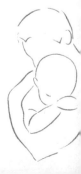

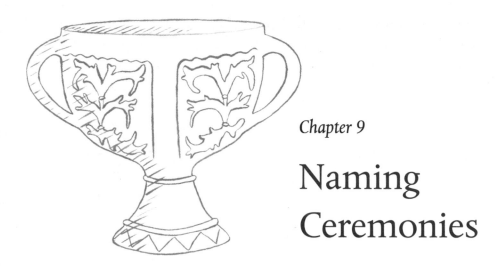

Chapter 9

Naming Ceremonies

"Everybody loves being welcomed by joyous, enthusiastic and happy faces when returning home from a long day of work or a trip away from home ... Being welcomed puts an end to our long journey. This is as close as I can explain the process of birth for souls coming to Earth: our children need to be joyfully welcomed when they are born."

Sobonfu Some[22]

"I definitely want Brooklyn to be christened, but I don't know into what religion yet."

David Beckham (quoted in The Mirror) 2002

The birth of a child is a miraculous event, a cause for celebration and, for those close to the child, the beginning of a life-long project. All over the world, ceremonies take place to give voice to the awe and thanksgiving that the safe delivery of a child inspires. These awaken the community to the practical and spiritual task of raising the child and supporting its parents. The bestowing of a name is usually a central part of that ceremony.

Sobonfu Some, in her book 'Welcoming Spirit Home', writes at length about the rituals for naming a child in her tribe in rural Burkino Faso. At around four months into the pregnancy there is a "hearing ritual" when elders gather to enquire of the incoming child what its life purpose is, why it is coming at this time and into this community. The mother goes into a trance and the child speaks through her. At this time a name is found that suits the life purpose communicated. Divinations are made to check with the ancestors that the name is approved, and it is kept secret. The first time the child's name is spoken aloud is at the naming ceremony, where the child is presented to the village. The elements and directions are called upon to bring blessing and protection. The grandmother or grandfather whispers the name to the child first, three times for a boy or four times for a girl, and then says it aloud the same number of times. Everyone present then comes near, whispers the name into the baby's ear, and speaks their blessings and hopes for the child.[23]

Although on the face of it this ritual is a far cry from a Church of England Christening, where a priest sprinkles holy water on a baby's forehead and, speaking his whole name aloud, makes the sign of a cross, perhaps the essential elements are not so different. In each case the child is presented to the tribe, orientated in his wider

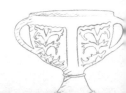

family, welcomed, blessed, named, and claimed by those to whom he belongs, and with whom he will share a belief system. There is something so ancient and universal in this ritual that people long for it, even when there is no church and no village that they really belong to any more.

Interestingly, the Church of England has recently devised a ceremony called "Thanksgiving for the Gift of a Child", offered since 1999, which recognises that many parents do not wish their child to be baptised but nevertheless, like the confused David Beckham, want to do something. (This service is described in more detail in Chapter 12, in the context of Adoption.) There are now even some local authorities offering civil baby naming ceremonies, rather in the way that civil marriages are carried out by an official Registrar. Humanists offer non-religious ceremonies, and have created a useful handbook on the subject.[24] There are also a growing number of pioneers who are finding new structures, borrowing from a wide range of traditions, and creating new naming ceremonies expressing their core beliefs in their own unique style. In this chapter I tell some of their stories. You will not find any 'off the peg' ceremony outlines here, for that would be missing the point. Instead I hope to demonstrate enough alternatives that you may be encouraged to do your own thing, be it a walk in the park with a few friends, or a large gathering with a ritual led by a celebrant. Two full stories of naming ceremonies are followed by a breakdown of the various elements that you might wish to consider when devising your own.

Heather's Naming

We organised a Naming Ceremony for Heather around her first birthday. We asked a celebrant to help us discern what we really wanted to say, and to hold the space for us. In two or three meetings and an exchange of emails, we worked out a shape. About 50 people, family and friends, gathered in our local village hall. We asked people to bring a flower, which was an amazingly simple and effective way to transform the space. One friend was in charge of vases, and was kept very busy receiving flowers and finding places for them all. Children were welcome to come but we had a crèche for little ones in a next-door room, in case they were bored and disruptive.

Our ceremony began with everyone singing Heather's favourite song at the time: 'Row, row, row your boat'. Then Phil read an extract about children from *The Prophet* by Kahlil Gibran and I performed a song I'd written for Heather. We wanted to do something to acknowledge Heather's ancestors, both to thank Phil's parents who had been very involved during Heather's first year, and to honour mine who were present only in spirit. We made an altar as the centrepiece of our circle. At the bottom was a soft cream baby blanket crocheted by Phil's mum, and a stone from a special valley where I go to meditate. On top were a bowl of water from the same valley, photos of both sides of the family (one of me as a baby at my Christening with mother, father and Grandmother), and a candle in my Grandmother's silver candlestick. I carried Heather with me as I went to light the candle, and she was very attentive as I showed her the picture and lit the candle.

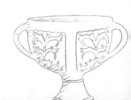

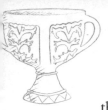

Then we introduced Heather's guide-parents. We had asked them all to bring something – be it an object or poem or little speech to put into the ceremony at this point. One had decided to dress as a fairy godmother for the occasion, and waved her 'wand' (a small white fishing net!) as she delivered blessings.

After this, in the focal point of the ceremony, I talked a little about why we had chosen Heather and Grace as her names and we invited everyone to join in saying, "Welcome, welcome, welcome Heather Grace." She was sprinkled with water from the valley, and Phil and I drank some too. We finished by singing 'We are' a song by Ysaye Maria Barnwell from Sweet Honey in the Rock: "For each child that's born, the morning star rises, and sings to the universe who we are."

All in all, it was a terribly emotional occasion, and not just for me. Very many people told me how moved they were. It seemed to touch some need in people to hear those things for themselves: that we are welcome here on the earth, that we are loved, blessed, cherished. The ceremony was made for Heather, but when we raised a glass we toasted all the children, and remembered that since we all start out as children, it included all the adults too.

We asked a friend to make a video of the event, principally because a couple of close family members weren't able to come, but it has been a lovely memento for us, and for Heather, who finds it fascinating.

Molly's Naming

Another Oxfordshire family made the River Thames the focus of their ceremony for their daughter Molly. This is her father's story:

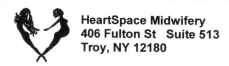

HeartSpace Midwifery
406 Fulton St   Suite 513
Troy, NY 12180

Colin: "We both wanted a ceremony for Molly, for us to recognise the fact that we had had a baby, and that she had reached life. We wanted to welcome her into the world, and into the community, but not push her into any religion. We're not very religious ourselves. We were too scared to go to the local vicar because we never go to church. We also wanted Molly to have god-parents. We did the ceremony on her first birthday.

I did some research on the Internet and found out about Humanist and Unitarian baby naming ceremonies and the Life Rites Association. I found a Native American blessing that we really liked, and some words from the Tao Te Ching. We also had readings from Francis Thompson and William Blake.

We live really near the river Thames, and have spent many happy hours swimming and hanging out on the bank. We wanted to have some physical symbol of welcoming Molly, and as water is a universal symbol of life, we decided that dunking her in the river would be a good welcome to our family.

About fifteen people came, family and friends. We made little origami boats and asked people to write their hopes and wishes on them for Molly. We walked down to the river and I talked a bit about what we were going to do and why. There were readings, and then we appointed the god-parents. They both spoke a little at that point. There was some music from some musical members of the family who had written a song for the occasion. Then I got into the water and launched all the little boats. They floated away, and got stuck in an eddy, so someone else helped to set them on their way again.

I took Molly and dunked her in the water, saying our words of welcome.

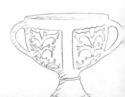

"We welcome you to the community of life and name you
Molly Rose Greaves.
May your days be full and long upon the earth.
May all be well with you in your journey through life.
We dedicate you to everything which is beautiful and truthful and
   good."

   I had felt a bit funny about doing it, but when the time came it
was fine. My mum said a short prayer, and we finished with a poem
by Spike Milligan, and some thank yous.

   When our second child Hannah came along, we did a similar
thing, but as we had invited more people to come, we couldn't
manage to make individual boats for everyone, so we made one
big boat, and everyone wrote their wishes on that. Also, Hannah
was much younger, so we only splashed water on her rather than
dunking her right in the river."

* * *

When to hold the Ceremony

In cultures where 'the village' makes rituals as a matter of daily life it
is possible to hold a ceremony in the early days after a birth, but in
our culture I wouldn't advise it. When getting to grips with looking
after a newborn babe you don't want to be thinking about hiring
the community centre and making cake. A first birthday works well
because it gives you time to think about god-parents, and gives a date
to aim for. Friends of mine who worked in a very rural and remote
part of northern Zimbabwe in the 1980s told me that people there
celebrate a child's arrival a year after the birth. There, it is taboo even

to mention the pregnancy, and the birth is not celebrated, but if the child survives the first precarious year, there is a celebration, and a gift is given to the person who delivered the child.

The Pagan festival of Imbolc, which comes on 2nd February and celebrates the first stirrings of spring, halfway between the winter solstice and the spring equinox, is a traditional time to give thanks for the safe arrival of children. Imbolc has two possible derivations. One, 'ImBolg' means literally 'in the belly' and suggests the first stirrings of spring happening invisibly underground in the belly of the earth. The other, 'Oimelc' means 'ewes milk' and refers to a celebration of the first lambs being born. If you have friends who have had babies in the last year, you could take this date as a time to get together for a joint celebration.

As with having a baby, there is no perfect time to have a naming ceremony. If you wait until you're completely ready and organised, it will never happen. Remember that it doesn't have to be complicated, and it doesn't have to be perfect; often the things that don't go according to plan are the best bits. And don't be afraid to ask for help. People get seized by the spirit of an event and will be honoured to take part.

Where to be

Since naming a child is a private ceremony with no legal significance, the only limits to where it can be held are those of comfort and practicality. Depending on the time of year and the number of people coming, it could happen at home, in a garden, a church hall, community centre, hillside, river's edge or beach. Sometimes a place

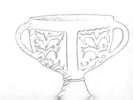

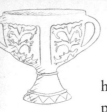

has a significance of its own and going to it with the child is a large part of the meaning of the event.

Naomi's family gathered to welcome her two sons on a piece of open heath land, with dramatic views over Devon, where six years earlier they had come to scatter the ashes of her grandmother. At that time, the place had recently been burnt, and so it was really 'ashes to ashes'. Now, the land was bright with vivid green gorse bushes, crowned with yellow flowers; a fitting backdrop for a contemplation of the new generation.

Chloe and Mark chose the garden of a church in the hills near their home in Herefordshire to welcome baby Rhys. It was important that there was a spring nearby, because they wanted to collect fresh water. For them, it was also important to be up high, for the views and the perspective that being nearer to the sky gives. Climbing the hill to the spring, climbing further to the church, then descending for tea in the town, and home for supper gave the shape of their day.

If the venue is a hall or community centre, it may need some warming up to be a really welcoming space. Even a fairly stark hall can be made cosy by hanging banners and bringing in flowers or branches. A selection of household angle-poise lights with some coloured bulbs is all you need to soften unsympathetic lighting.

You could ask all the guests to bring something to decorate the space. This is a good way to transform a space easily without asking too much of any one person. People could bring balloons, streamers, mobiles, flowers, plants, fabric, pictures etc. If you do this, you need to factor in time to hang things at the start of your event. A variation on this idea is to ask people to bring a decoration that expresses something they love about the world, or something they would wish for the child.

Special Clothes

In a Jewish ceremony, the baby is sometimes wrapped in a prayer shawl that was used at the parents' wedding. In my own family there is a Christening robe that has been passed down from my father's side of the family. Recently my niece was christened in this intricate white cotton robe and it was an extraordinary thought that some of the lanky teenagers and their parents standing round the font had once been the baby in the robe. My father died as quite a young man, at a time when I was the new baby. Now I was holding my niece in the robe that I knew he'd once worn. It brought the ancestors nearer.

Opening the Ceremony

Coming together from many places, and long journeys, people need a little time to settle before the ceremony, preparing the mind to be in a receptive and unhurried state. A walk to the site of the ceremony can shake off the stresses of the journey, and this can be made into a procession by carrying flags, or if it is dusky, lanterns. This is a great way to involve children, who can make the decorations.[25]

Jessica and Stephen invited people at the opening of their gathering to keep a silence and meditate on "The Child". They found that while the children and infants present weren't able to keep the silence, their cries and words became part of the meditation. Eddie and Sarah took people on a walking meditation around their garden before they settled together on rugs on the lawn.

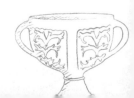

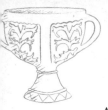

Introduction

An introduction is needed to welcome the guests, and explain what is about to happen and why. Aunt Mabel may not have been to anything like this before, and may be reassured by some basic information. If you have printed an order of service, which I think is an excellent idea, you can ask people to look at this as you go through it.

Colin and Alison wrote these words:

"We have chosen, as do many parents nowadays, not to have Molly baptised into any formal religion. We would prefer her to make up her own mind as to which, if any, spiritual path is right for her when she reaches adulthood. We would however like to celebrate her naming with friends and family, which is why, albeit somewhat much later than we really should have, we are all here today for a joint celebration of her naming and the huge step of her reaching the ripe old age of ONE. There is no official value to this naming ceremony, other than the value we give to it; its meaning is no more and no less than the meaning we have chosen to place upon it, but we would hope that one day Molly will be pleased to discover that we welcomed her arrival with thoughtfulness, as well as with festivity."

Readings

"You were the wished-for one,
the gift that nested in my heart,
like a bird, a soft kiss, a murmur."

Jeannie Donald

Whether you favour Spike Milligan or Silvia Plath, when it comes to finding poems or other readings there is no shortage of material to choose from. It could be something that expresses the delight of a new baby, or that speaks of the divine duties of the parents. Going in search of the perfect poem, leafing through poetry books in the library, asking friends, scanning the Internet for ideas can be a pleasure in itself. Poems and sourcebooks I particularly recommend browsing in can be found in the Resources section.

Songs

Songs can be wonderful, or difficult, depending on how your family and friends feel about singing. What is needed are songs that people know, or that are very easy to pick up. Given that it is an event for a baby, a very simple lullaby or child's song could be appropriate.

Jessica: "We sang a little lullaby that we had made up for Leyla and everyone joined in. It's just her name repeated over and over, and it's something she's heard regularly from the earliest days. It was lovely hearing everyone sing it."

Megan is from a Welsh family of keen singers, so songs were an important part of the naming of her son. "We chose songs with strong imagery. There was one about a river, which was chosen because of his name, Jordon, and another Celtic blessing song, 'Deep Peace'. I've sung him those particular songs a lot since the ceremony and I hope that something goes in."

If you would like to sing something but can't find the right song, you may know someone who would enjoy writing something very simple. If communal singing would just make everyone feel awkward, then listening to live or recorded music may be a better option.

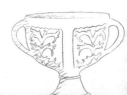

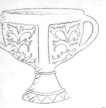

Making Pledges

Some parents like to make explicit the commitments they are giving their children by making a pledge. These can be very short and pithy, like this one written by Megan and Thomas and spoken together:

"We make a lifelong commitment to supporting you physically, emotionally and spiritually to the best of our abilities. We commit to nurturing your growth, while respecting your freedom of choice."

Other people's are more lyrical. These extracts are from longer individual speeches by Eddie and Sarah to their one-year-old son:

"I promise to try always to be there for you, like a rocky islet in the foaming Atlantic swells; so that however far we may be swept apart by the currents, I will still be there when the tide turns."

"Let us enjoy life, look out for each other and laugh together. Let's also remember to let each other change and evolve. When times are tough and the road is rocky, let us remember love is the source and strength of all things."

The commitment from the parents can be accompanied by prayers for guidance and support from spirit, as in these words spoken by Chloe and Mark:

"We commit to be there for Rhys and to support him. We acknowledge his descent from the spiritual realms, and the purpose that lay behind this, which is yet to be known. We ask that we may be guided to enable and empower that purpose in order that it be made manifest."

Reinventing God-parents

Mentors, spiritual parents, god-parents, lay-parents, guardians, guardian angels, guard-parents, guide-parents, supporting adults… whatever you choose to call them, these are people that parents ask to take a particularly close role in their child's life.

For some people this is specifically a spiritual role, for others it is more a case of asking other adults to complement the parents' strengths and weaknesses. Given that we live in a world of small family units and many one-parent families, there can be real value in forging an extended family by invitation.

Sarah and Eddie took a particularly creative approach to appointing god-parents by spelling out the areas of life they wanted them to take care of for their boy. Thus a nature-loving friend was given responsibility for nurturing the 'the outdoors' in Alistair's life. A city-living friend was charged with looking after 'art and culture'. They also chose someone to look after 'the fun side of life' and someone 'to nurture his spiritual development'.

As they said, "Some of these overlap, and we chose the people first rather than the roles we thought they should fill, so we don't intend the roles to be formal or constricting, but more of a help and a guide. Being a god-parent could involve taking Alistair away for a weekend camping or inviting him to the cinema, but the main thing is to be part of his life, make him laugh and feel valued."

Each friend was asked to prepare some words to give at the ceremony about their own wishes for and promises to the child. They also decided to invite all the god-parents together again in five year's time to revisit their pledges.

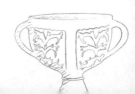

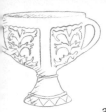

Jessica and Stephen also took a novel and good-humoured approach to the appointing of god-parents. They decided that, as bringing up a child was a testing task, they would hold a mock "tournament" to test the abilities of the prospective god-parents. They invited them for a weekend camping, and asked each person to bring a challenge to set the others. Chief amongst these was to pack a tent away in its carrying bag in a certain time span, a feat that the parents themselves found impossible. The god-parents, duly appointed, agreed to go camping again together in a year's time. Incidentally, this appointing of god-parents happened on Kai's first birthday, some time after his naming ceremony, which is a good reminder that modern ceremony is infinitely flexible.

Naming the Child

Although some people have a welcoming ceremony for their child that does not include naming, in most cases saying the child's full name aloud is a central event in the ritual. Our name, and the story of our name, is an indelible legacy from our parents. Even if we change our name later in life, that too is part of our story. So in naming a child we bear a great responsibility. A name affirms both the unique identity of an individual, and also the family or tribe to which he or she belongs.

At a naming ceremony, people often talk about why certain names were chosen. They might be keeping alive the memory of an ancestor or honouring a living relative. They might be chosen for a particular meaning or association.

Liz: "It's been joyful to see both our children connect with their names and become rooted in them. We didn't name them lightly.

I like being able to give good answers to the why questions, when they ask. I chose Rowan because of my good associations with the tree – like the fact that it thrives in difficult situations. Adam chose Laurie because as a boy he was passionate about the writing of Laurie Lee. So for each of them there is a link back to something that their parents valued and hoped to pass on, and they know that."

The moment of naming the child is usually the high point of the ceremony. Sometimes the climax is expressed by lifting the child high, raising voices and perhaps releasing something into the air, along with our high hopes. Here are some examples:

"Welcome to your life here on earth. We are so glad you have come to us. You, who have already travelled far through doorways of the soul." Karen Kay

"Welcome Thomas, enjoy your life!"
"Welcome Joseph, enjoy your life!"
Thomas's helium balloon whirled out on a gust of wind, and, moments later, Joseph's balloon raced after it, both quickly rising above the hill and disappearing into the sky beyond. It was a fittingly vigorous welcome to two boys into a family of spirited adventurers.

At a joint naming ceremony for seven children of various ages prepared by artists from Welfare State International a rocket was fired into the sky with each name as these words were called to the winds:

"May their names sing as long as these brave trees!
May their lives echo on in the stars!

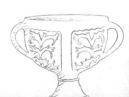

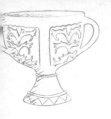

May our love give them help as they travel alone!
May our prayers hold their hand as they fly!"[26]

Anointing with Water

Splashing the child's head with water or immersing her fully is a more traditional way to mark a naming.

Following old Celtic instincts, Chloe and Mark took flowers to decorate the well where they collected water for their son's naming. Their pilgrimage to the well was a way of honouring the spirit of nature in her life-giving flow. They carried the water and shared it amongst them all as a purification, in their preparation for the task of parenting, and as an affirmation of their connection to each other and to the source of life. Each person touched the head of the child with the water, by way of blessing.

Jessica and Stephen used water that a friend had brought back from a sacred mountain in Tibet. "Stephen and I had both wanted to make the pilgrimage to Mount Kailash, but neither of us have done it yet. We named Kai after the mountain, and maybe he's become our daily pilgrimage. It felt right to bless him with the water from that special place."

In his book *From Beginning to End*, Robert Fulghum tells about a couple who saved rainwater from the rainy camping holiday when they conceived their first child. The father kept the water to toast his partner, if she should conceive, and they also kept some to anoint the child.

Planting a Tree

Sacred to our ancestors, the tree is a universal symbol of life, with its roots in the matter of the world and its branches stretching to the heavens. Given that each human will use the resources from many trees in its lifetime (the average American uses the equivalent of nine mature pine trees each year, just for paper), what better to do on the arrival of a child than plant a tree?[27]

If the time of year for your ceremony is autumn or winter, planting a tree can be carried out as part of the event, and the group of people can get involved. You could either gather to hold your whole ceremony in the place where the tree is to be planted, or go there afterwards.

Jessica: "When we planted our tree an unexpected thing happened – other people threw things in the hole too – leaves and things – as blessings. Then everyone stamped the earth down around it."

Planting a tree may be prompted by the desire to give the child a connection to a place where he can go to remember his roots. In a mobile society, this is easier said than done. We rarely have easy access to land where planting a tree would be appropriate, and we don't often stay in the same place long enough to see a tree grow to maturity. Still, even if the child cannot visit his own tree throughout his life, making an early relationship of this kind may well awaken in him a capacity to connect with nature at other times and in other places.

If there is a place you like to go walking, try asking permission to plant a tree from the landowner. They may be agreeable, especially if it is privately owned. National Trust, English Heritage or Forestry Commission land will have policies about what and where and when trees are planted, and it may be harder to get what you would like, but it is worth asking.

Do bear in mind that trees need to be planted carefully, watered deeply and protected from deer and other creatures while they are

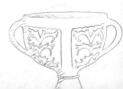

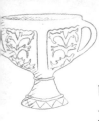

becoming established. It can be difficult if the symbolic tree dies. If you like the symbolism of planting a tree, but not the practical work of looking after it, a local Arboretum may have a 'tree adoption' scheme, where you can pay a donation for them to put a plaque on a young sapling. Or you could send a donation to the Woodland Trust (see Resources), who will plant a tree in your name, and send you a certificate.

Alternatively, if you have a garden, you could plant something there. It could be bulbs that flower on the child's birthday, or a rose bush; a time-honoured symbol of the joy and the pain of life. Megan and Thomas planted a Wisteria tree in their garden when they named their son, who is now five years old. They enjoy watching him take care of it and take pride in seeing it grow. "Look at my plant!" he says, as he carefully fills a watering can in the dry summer months.

Blessings

After the climax of the ceremony, it is natural that the assembled company will want to add their good wishes and blessings. This can be done very simply, with a few words, or dramatised in any number of creative ways, which are good for involving other children, like the floating boats in Molly's story. Rice or petals can be thrown into the air for good luck, while everyone shouts something like, "Blessings and Joy!"

In Gaelic tradition, the child would be passed around the circle of well-wishers and each in turn would speak their wishes for the child directly to him. The direction of the passing was sun-wise, to make a connection with the rhythm and cycle of the seasons. Megan and Thomas adapted this idea by carrying their son around the circle of guests and asking each of them to say something that they loved about the world that he was entering. At the close of their ceremony, other children softly blew bubbles around him while the adults sang the chorus of an Incredible String Band song: "May the long-time sun shine upon you".

Freya, aged four, was welcomed at a druid ceremony, and she remembers walking around the circle of friends and receiving words and gifts from each of them. I asked her about this when she was ten (going on 16) and she proudly went to get her box to show me. In it were a pendant and a stone from this event, amongst other childhood treasures, including a letter from the tooth fairy and her first bus ticket. The little spontaneous gifts of stones and necklaces have become sacred objects that remind her of the people who gave them, and, together with her other significant objects, tell something of the story of her life.

Here are three traditional blessings.

An African Blessing

A little lemon is touched to the baby's lips, with the words, "Sometimes life is bitter."
A little honey is touched to the baby's lips: "Sometimes life is sweet"
A little wine is touched to the baby's lips: "But always, it is up to you to make it joyful." The wine is shared, and the community make a commitment to support the child to make life joyful.

An Irish Blessing

May the road rise with you,
May the wind be ever at your back,

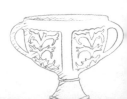

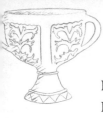

May the sun shine warm upon your face,
May the rain fall soft upon your fields,
And until we meet again,
May God/Love hold you
In the hollow of his/her hand.

A Jewish Blessing
"May this little one, (name) be big!"

Sharing a Cup of Celebration

A horn of mead, a silver chalice of wine, a bowl of spring-water or a magnum of champagne – raising a vessel to life and sharing it amongst friends is one of our oldest ways of marking kinship and friendship. Sometimes this happens in a more informal way, along with the cutting of a cake, and toasts to the parents and child. Other times it is a part of the ceremony.

Jessica: "When Kai was born a relative who lives in Scotland sent a present of a 'Quaich' – a little silver 'Cup of Welcome' from the Highlands. I think they use it for whisky when guests arrive, but we used it in our ceremony for the spring water to bless Kai and to share amongst us."

These words were used as a ritual created by the Society for Humanistic Judaism:

"This cup of wine is the cup of life. It is the symbol of a family and the sign of continuity from generation to generation. Rena is more than an individual. She is part of the chain of life that stretches from the past into the future. Let us raise this cup to life"[28]

Following this idea, a cup is sometimes given as a gift to the child, expressing the hope that he, as a new member of the community, will share the cup of life with others, in hospitality and in friendship. In pre-Christian Europe, a child would be named after a renowned kinsman. In a ritual called 'Wetting the Baby's Head', water was sprinkled on the child's head, and the kinsman would give the child a cup called a 'name fastening' cup.

Closing

Once the child is named and blessed, the business of this ceremony is over. The closing part might include another prayer or song, but all that really needs to be communicated is thanks to everyone for coming and, usually, an invitation to the festivities to come.

Festivities

With the ceremony over, it is time for feasting and relaxing. To keep costs down, you could ask your friends to bring their favourite dish to share. Symbolically, this is an act of exchange that is the stuff of community, and practically, swapping recipes is a great icebreaker.

Before the guests leave, you might ask them to write in a special book, sign a certificate to keep a record of who was there to witness the naming, or make a wish on a 'wishing tree'. To make a Wishing Tree, take a good-sized branch and bed it solidly into a pot of earth or stones. Provide ready cut-out shapes with ties of string, wool or ribbon. These can be parcel labels, or you can be more creative and make leaves, stars, angels or any shape you like. Also provide plenty of pens. Write a wish or a blessing on a 'leaf' and tie it on the tree. People will get the idea!

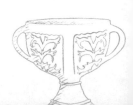

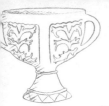

Gifts

People like to bring gifts to a party, and that can be delightful, but there are only so many toys, mobiles and quickly outgrown clothes a baby needs, and maybe you would prefer to stimulate thoughtfulness rather than consumerism amongst your friends and family.

One alternative is to ask people to bring a poem they like to stick into a scrapbook, creating an eclectic anthology for the child to enjoy in future years. Or it could be a picture postcard, resulting in a personalised picture book. Another idea is for everyone to bring a photograph of themselves to put in an album, so the child has a reference point for friends and family she may not see regularly. Or it could be a favourite recipe, so that in days to come she can make 'Liz's chocolate cake' or 'Auntie Anne's coconut curry.' For all of these ideas, you need to give people some notice, and record it on the invitation.

To make a special present for the future, ask guests to bring something little, with a note attached, then place these in a box to be sealed and opened on an 18th or 21st birthday. Sealed letters are also a wonderful way to send a goodwill message into the future. They could be read out at the ceremony and then sealed and kept safe until a future date.

Naomi asked her family and friends to bring a symbolic gift, and the giving of these was part of the actual ceremony. People interpreted the idea very widely, but in all cases it brought extra meaning to the presents, and provided a relaxed way in which people could say a few words about what was meaningful to them. The boys' grandfather gave postcards of gig racing on the Isles of Scilly. He explained that pilots would row out to meet the incoming ships at the mouth of harbour and compete for the business of guiding them safely in. He drew an analogy with the boys needing good guidance in their early lives, and he also wished them the fun of competition. Another relative gave the child a towel, and read the extract from Douglas Adams' *A Hitch-Hiker's Guide to the Galaxy* where he says that anyone who can hitchhike across the galaxy and still have a towel is a man to be admired. He hoped that Thomas would grow to be a man who 'really knew where his towel was'.

If you have asked people not to bring presents, you could organise a collection for a charity that benefits children, and spread the goodwill from your event to the wider world in a very practical way.

Thank-you Gifts

It sometimes feels appropriate to give something to everyone who has come to celebrate the naming, or to a few people who have played an important role. At Heather's ceremony we had so many flowers that we could re-distribute them to our helpers. I've seen children very much appreciate a slab of chocolate with the name of the new child and the date of the naming piped on it in icing. And perhaps not only the children…

* * *

Organising a naming ceremony does take time and effort, but I think the stories in this chapter show how it can be both creative and satisfying. For the parents it provides a strong foundation for future parenting, as they have to agree and publicly express what they deem most important, and discover how the tone and style of their family will express itself. In holding a public event the parents

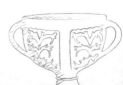

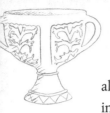

also have the opportunity to invite the participation of particular individuals and the whole 'village' in the shared joys and trials of bringing up a child.

I also believe that a naming ceremony brings great benefit for the child. One thing many people have told me is how the baby seems to be especially alert at the time of his naming, apparently conscious at some level of the loving attention directed towards him. Heather certainly seemed to blossom after her ceremony, becoming ever more confident and ebullient as she learnt to walk and talk.

Marking the major rites of passage – including the arrival of a child – is very important for the community too. If we skip them because they are too difficult, too expensive, because the family is too far-flung, or we are not sure what we believe in anyway, we are denying ourselves the very occasions that make life rich, and leave the strongest impressions in our shared memories. I never cease to be amazed by what beauty a team of people with a unified purpose can create. The arrival of a child is such a joyful cause for a celebration; let us not hold back in creating occasions worthy of its inspiration!

Chapter 10

Miscarriage

Miscarriage is a death in the heart of life, a death that happens inside the body of a woman. Sometimes a child just brushes the earth lightly, and is gone before the embryo is anything more than a few cells. Even so, there may already have been a strong connection, love, the beginning of hopes and dreams for the child. Later in a pregnancy, when the being has made itself known through kicks and a visible bump, a whole community may have already begun to make a place for it. Whenever a miscarriage happens, it is a loss that cuts deeply, and needs to be grieved.

Medically speaking, a miscarriage is defined as the death of a foetus of less than 24 weeks gestation. At this age the foetus has no status as a person in law, and therefore a burial or cremation is not required. However, many people are finding that a funeral of some kind is exactly what is needed at an emotional level. A good ritual can hold in a symbolic form both the deep letting go that needs to be done at this time, and also an honouring of whatever blessing the brief pregnancy brought. It can support a woman, or a couple, through the desolation of thwarted life, and back into a remembrance of beauty and love.

Burial

If it is possible to honour the actual remains of an unborn child by burial, this can be very helpful. The Celts called the spirits of unborn or stillborn children 'mac talla' meaning 'rock-child' or 'echo'. The foetus would have been returned to the wild, buried after dark in a sacred place, where the spirit would have a safe place to rest.[29]

Abbey: "I miscarried three times, and each time I caught the foetus with my hands. My hands were there without me thinking, but I'm very glad I did that. The foetus was like a kidney bean. As it started to cool down, I wanted to wrap it up. The letting go is already beginning then, as the warmth leaves it. The first one I just wrapped in tissue paper, put plastic around it and placed in my pocket. I couldn't leave it behind. This happened on the same day as my mother's funeral. Later that day I went with my partner and we dug a tiny hole under a tree in the cemetery and tucked it under a stone. We collected a few of my mother's flowers and put them there on the little grave.

The second time I caught the foetus over a chamber pot and put it in a Tupperware container in the freezer, because I was still cramping a lot and not ready to go out yet. A couple of days later we walked in a forest until we found a place we liked. We dug a grave, lined it with leaves and pretty things we found, laid the foetus in and covered it with leaves. We sang songs and cried and prayed together. We talked to the baby, saying goodbye, go now, you're free

The third time I miscarried at eleven weeks. We buried the foetus in the garden and planted a bush on top of it. We were too exhausted to go anywhere else."

Lucy: "When my first child Ash was two I had a miscarriage. When you miscarry, the body has already broken its ties with the baby, but I'd already put this child into my family in my imagination. That was what was hard to break. When Ash was born we kept the placenta and had meant to bury it and plant a tree, but two years had passed and it was still in the freezer! We decided to bury the placenta together with the few blood clots from the miscarried child in a spot under a chestnut tree near the canal where we live. Andy dug a hole, we read some poems and just talked to the child, saying how sorry we were that it couldn't stay because we would have loved to know it, and thanking it for the love it had brought in its brief time with us. When our cat died we buried her in the same place. I have this image of the two children playing conkers and three-legged Puss playing with them.

I had a second miscarriage nearly a year later. This time Ash was old enough to understand a little about why we were sad. We were singing songs, and he suggested we could sing Postman Pat to the baby. So we did that too; that was his contribution."

Symbolic Burial

Sometimes it is not possible to bury the actual remains of the child. If the miscarriage happens in a hospital, the remains may be taken away before you have begun to think about asking for them, or you might wish to mark a miscarriage that happened some time ago. In this case, a burial of something symbolic of the baby can be performed instead, as in the following story, where Isobel found inspiration from a Japanese ritual practice.

Isobel: "I had been in Japan for two months with a new boyfriend, when I discovered I was pregnant. The same day it became clear that it was an ectopic pregnancy, and suddenly I was a medical emergency. I had an operation in a Japanese hospital that left me traumatised, exhausted and two thousand pounds in debt. The doctors showed me the tiny embryo in a metal kidney dish. It was half the size of my fingernail. Still, I knew it had been alive before the operation, and was now dead.

Months later we went up to Koyasan, a mountain top settlement near Osaka. Walking in the forest of cypress trees we came upon a bridge over a river, where unborn children are remembered. There are statues along the side of the river representing gods who are believed to watch over children after they die, and guard them in the other world. You can pour water over the statues and pray to them. I remember asking that they take care of my child, and that it would know it was loved.

There are monks by the river and you can go and ask them to inscribe a piece of bamboo with the name of the lost child. The monks write the name in beautiful calligraphy and the sticks are left in the river until the inscription is washed away, and can no longer be read. I did this each autumn for three years, and after that, I didn't need to do it any more.

Years later in England, I miscarried again. Again I was rushed to hospital and had a four-hour labour, which was very painful. I had thought of the baby as Leo or Leonie, because I knew it would be born in early July, in the sign of Leo. When July came, my partner and I were separating, but we had already arranged to go away together that weekend to the coast. I knew that the due date would be a hard day to get through, so, probably inspired by the Japanese rituals, I thought of doing something symbolic.

I had a little wooden sculpture of a woman and a baby, which a sculptor had made for me in Japan, and I brought it with me. I talked to Julian about it being the due date for the baby, and once we started talking, he recognised that he too had a need to do something. We just walked to the end of the cob with the little doll. In the statue the woman and child were naked, so we found seaweed and wrapped them up in black and red strands. Then we cast them into the ocean.

There weren't any particular words. I wanted to talk to the child, but I felt I didn't know the language. They were in a different world. Ritual seemed to be easier than talking.

On the way back from the beach we went to an aquarium and there were Mermaid's Purses in an illuminated tank. We could see the little dogfish swimming around in the purse, and they, like us, have a nine-month gestation period. Something about that completed the ritual for me: it felt hopeful to see new life.

I was very glad to have done something to remember the child and let it go. Afterwards I felt I could place the experience and set it

down. It settled somewhere on that sea bed, and came down to rest somewhere in me."

All the women above felt a need to communicate with the child as part of their ritual. If speaking aloud does not seem possible, writing a letter may be easier. This could be buried with the remains, or burnt.

Remembering the Child

Some people have found they wanted something to keep for themselves to remember the child by. Something small but precious such as a ring or a locket might feel right. If, like me, you are good at losing jewellery, you might feel happier with a picture for the house or statue in the garden.

Browsing online, I even found a website where you could place a star in a virtual sky to represent your child. I was touched by the sheer number of stars there, with names in many languages. There is surely some comfort in knowing that, however little talked about miscarriage is, it is an experience shared by a great many women the world over.

Isobel's story above shows that there is sometimes a need to repeat a ritual a number of times before the wound is healed. As with any grief, the pain is likely to take time to abate, and in years to come the anniversaries, both of the miscarriage date and the due date, may be times when emotions are strongly felt. A small ritual at these times such as lighting a candle, bringing in some flowers and spending a little time in reflection would make the date conscious, and possibly prevent the hard feelings from spilling into the rest of your life.

An Outline for a Miscarriage Ritual

In this very delicate ritual, it is not necessary to use words at all but, for those who find it helpful to have a script, I offer the following text as a starting point. This ritual could be used whether the burial is actual or symbolic. If you find you have already begun thinking of the child's name, you can use this in the burial. If not, you could just find a term of endearment, such as Little One.

If possible, find a companion to witness your ritual. It might be the father of the miscarried foetus, or a trusted friend. Decide where you can go to make a burial, either of the actual remains or a symbolic object of your choice, for example a stone or a stick, which you could wind wool around. It might be a garden or a place in nature, but make sure it is somewhere, or at a time of day, when you are not likely to be overlooked or disturbed. A simpler alternative would be to release something into a river or the sea, and not to plant anything.

Opening Prayer: Spirit of Life, you are present in all things, in my body, in all things living and growing and changing today. Yet this little one that came to us is no longer living and growing. Our hearts are broken because we already loved her. We felt in her all the power and potential of new life, and yet she didn't come through to meet us.

Addressing the child: Little One (or child's name), we would have made a place for you in our family. We already had dreams of what we would do together (name some...) We let you go now. Be free. Go well on your journey, wherever that may take you.

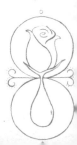

Burial: Set down the remains, or your symbolic object in the site you have chosen.

Addressing the child: You are gone from us, but in your short life you brought many blessings (name some, perhaps scattering flowers as you do so). We thank you for these.

Either: You will always have a place in our hearts. We remember you with this symbol (e.g. a necklace or ring).

And / Or: This child is gone, but life continues. We sow these bulbs / plant this bush as a sign of our faith in life.

Poem: e.g. Christina Rossetti's 'Come to me in the Silence of the Night'

Closing Prayer: Spirit of Life, hold us through this time of sadness. We ask for healing for ourselves, for our bodies and for our hearts. Help us to accept what we cannot understand, and bring us, in time, back into the light of hopefulness.

* * *

There is great eloquence in the stories in this chapter of how women have dealt with miscarriages. Whilst the stories are all sad, the overwhelming feeling one is left with is love and tenderness. The work of grieving a miscarriage is nothing to be ashamed of, and doesn't need to be borne alone. The tears shed are not for nothing. As a friend of mine wrote in a song, "Tears are the prayers and the meditations of woman."

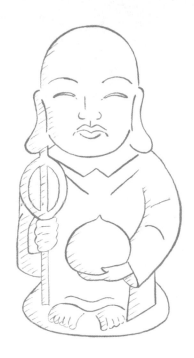

Chapter 11

Stillbirth

S ometimes, for reasons known or mysterious, a baby dies in
the womb when it is well on its way to becoming fully formed.
A mother must labour to bring her baby into the world, but
the joyful cries of birth are cruelly replaced by the silence of death.
There can be no easy route through the pain and shock of this
experience: how profoundly sad to be preparing for a funeral, when
a celebration of birth has been expected.

Yet, as the stories in this chapter show, it is possible to handle
even this experience with care, courage and a sense of rightness.
When the world seems upside down, there is comfort in listening to
your intuition and arranging things as you see fit. An honest facing
up to the death, a natural burial and a funeral that contains the
individual loss within the universal round of life and death – these
things can begin to restore a sense of order.

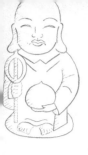

Spending Time with the Stillborn Baby

Happily, hospitals today are far more understanding than they used to be about the value for bereaved parents of spending time with their stillborn baby. In the past it was common for the bodies of stillborn children to be taken away and disposed of by the hospital, and countless women suffered the ache to hold and tend to the baby they had laboured to birth. Nowadays, parents are free to spend as much time with their baby as they need and may wash and dress the child after birth, take photographs, and even take the stillborn baby home.

Liz Rothschild gave birth to a stillborn girl at five months.

Liz: "We wanted to carry her home in a basket, but the hospital staff felt she should be transported secretly, in a sealed container. Clearly to them she represented a piece of medical failure. I persisted, and eventually was allowed to do as I wished. We wrapped her in a white child's sheet. She looked like a tiny baby, with thin skin. Our other two children were given the choice whether to hold her or not. Our son, aged 6, did hold her, but my 8 year old daughter decided not to."

Mary Wallace lost two children in the womb.

Mary: "When John was born, the hospital supported us to see and hold him. In the case of Alex, we took him home for a few days before the funeral. My other children, both under seven years old at the time, also saw and held their little brothers and were filled with wonderment and awe at their beauty and perfection. We took black and white photographs of the babies. It seemed an odd thing to do, but I was very glad we did. I had them on display in my living room for a while. They were not easy to look at, but it was very important to me to have them."

On the subject of photographs, *The Guardian* reported that a father of a very damaged stillborn baby had a photograph taken of just the baby's fingers curled around his hand.[30]

There may already have been a name associated with this child. If not, giving the child a name can help to frame the experience and make it easier to talk about. It also seems wise not to save this name for another child that might come in the future.

Burial or Cremation and Funerals

A stillborn baby older than 24 weeks must legally be buried or cremated. Hospitals will help to arrange a burial or cremation according to the parents' wishes, unless the parents decide to organise it themselves. Many cemeteries and crematoria have a particular place for babies, and in some cases do not charge for their services. When considering cremation, be aware that a tiny baby's body may leave no ashes to scatter.

There is no legal obligation to hold a funeral at all, and no restrictions on how this might take place.

Mary Wallace: "My husband found solace in making beautiful coffins for each of the babies out of pine. It was something he had the skills to do, and was very comforting for him, at a time when so much was outside of his control. We lined the coffins with a quilted fabric and laid the babies there, wrapped in a little shawl. We went out as a family and chose little gifts from each of us to put in the coffin – a butterfly brooch, a carved wooden heart, little toys.

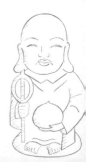

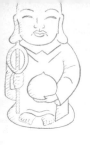

Neither my husband nor myself are religious at all, but we were lucky to have a wonderful hospital chaplain who supported us in making the funeral, without enquiring into our beliefs. He read some words from the Bible, but it was his presence that was important to us rather than his words. The babies are buried next to each other in a rose garden especially for infants in one of the city cemeteries. At the graveside ceremony we both read a piece of poetry and threw flowers onto the coffin. We said goodbye, and we have sad but lovely memories.

Snowdrops had a particular significance for us at that time as a symbol of purity and innocence. We made an announcement of birth/death card, which had a line drawing of snowdrops on it. Every year when the snowdrops come up it's a lovely reminder."[31]

Since the experience of her babies' deaths, Mary Wallace has become a celebrant with the Humanist Society of Scotland and now conducts non-religious funerals, including ceremonies for babies and children. One of the things she sometimes offers is a basket of sprigs of evergreen, which people cast into the grave. Evergreen is symbolic of the undying love with which the child is held in the hearts of those who knew him or her.

At the time of their daughter's stillbirth, Liz Rothschild was already working as a celebrant, helping people to mark the significant stages of their lives with ceremonies. Since she and her husband live on a farm with a large garden, it felt natural to bury the baby themselves, and to involve the children.

"We buried Cara in a bank in the garden, and placed a round stone on top. We read a poem, and planted forget-me-nots nearby – that was the children's choice."

The law permits up to four burials on private land without planning permission. It is generally advisable, though not legally necessary, to check with the local Environment Agency first. They are unlikely to have any objections provided that the grave is not within ten metres of any standing or running water, or 50 metres of a well, borehole or spring that supplies water for human consumption. More information is available from the Natural Death Centre.[32]

Memories and Anniversaries

As with all losses, the grieving process takes time, and anniversaries are likely to be times when feelings rise to the surface. Marking this time as a family by looking at photographs together or taking flowers to the grave gives space to feelings and prevents them from sabotaging the rest of life.

Mary: "One of the things that helped me was making a memory box. I got a flat-packed storage box, covered it in paper, and filled it with special things. There were handprints and footprints from the hospital, the identification wristband that never went on him, notes from the birth, photographs, and little gifts that people gave us at the time."

Children who Grieve

The loss of a baby often affects children who have begun to be excited about the arrival of a new sibling. It may well be a child's first experience of death, and it will certainly be a significant time, which needs to be sensitively handled.

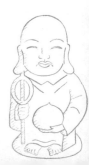

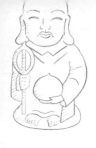

People understandably want to shield young children from the reality of death, but the fantasy that a child may create to fill the gap of unknowing may be much worse than the reality. Where there is openness, the child learns that he can trust his parents to tell him the truth, and can be comforted from nightmares by the knowledge that things are only as bad as they are.

It is important to give children choices in matters such as whether they want to see or hold the stillborn baby. Mary's young son was inquisitive about all aspects of his sibling's death and burial. After the funeral he drew a picture of the graveyard, clearly showing bodies in the coffins under the ground.

One kindergarten class were invited to take part in the funeral of a stillborn child, who was the sibling of one of the class. As a group they painted the little cardboard coffin for the baby. What better way to receive your first lesson in death than through gentle community involvement like this? It normalises the experience of bereavement which, after all, is a very natural part of life.

* * *

My heart goes out to anyone who has to cope with the stillbirth of their child. When something like this happens, we have a choice about whether to retreat from life and grow bitter, or whether to fully accept the experience, and deepen into life through it. I am very grateful to the contributors in this chapter, Mary and Liz, both of whom clearly chose the latter path, and reached a place where they could offer support to other people in times of loss.

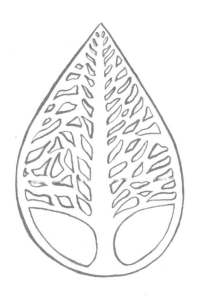

Chapter 12

Adoption

*"They told me I'd forget you, instead
I hid you in the crevices of my heart so
I wouldn't."*[33]

A doption is a complex and sensitive arrangement, which brings life-long gains and challenges for all the parties involved. The only official ritual of the adoption process is the court order, when parental responsibility for a child is legally transferred to the adoptive parent(s). Yet there are many more moments where the emotional needs of those affected by the adoption could be well served by a ritual. This chapter offers ideas for rituals for birth parents who have lost a child to adoption, for adoptive parents, and for adopted children.

The term adoption covers a great many different situations, and by no means all of these are covered in this chapter. The person adopting may be single or part of a couple, heterosexual or same sex. The child being adopted may be a baby, a child or a young person, from this country or from far away. Sometimes a step-parent adopts a child when he or she gets married, so the marriage takes on a family

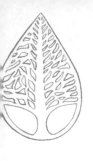

joining theme. Sometimes one part of a lesbian couple legally takes parental responsibility for their partner's birth child, although this is becoming less necessary now that Civil Partnerships are possible. Each adoption is as unique as all the individuals involved, but I hope the material here may be useful as a basis for tailoring ceremonies to suit all kinds of situations.

When considering using any of these ideas with children, great sensitivity needs to be used in discerning what is best for the child. Some children would be happy to be the focus of attention at a ceremony; others are shy and would panic at the very idea. Yet, the predictable structure of a ritual, with calm, unhurried time, good attention and honest compassionate talking, can be very stabilising for a child. Initial apprehension can turn to enthusiasm if the child realises that her ideas and contributions are used and appreciated in the ceremony. Other children in the family need just as much careful inclusion.

For Birth Parents

Since the 1926 Adoption Act, at which time adoption was seen as a panacea for many of society's ills, an estimated three quarters of a million women have parted with a child for adoption. Mothers who gave up a child for adoption used to be told they would forget all about it. They didn't. Many of them are still hoping against hope that they will be reunited with their grown-up adopted child.

These days, women are much less likely to see adoption as the answer to an unwanted pregnancy. More commonly, it is older children who are taken into care because the family is not coping, and the children are deemed to be at risk. Social Services will try to support the birth mother to keep the children as far as possible. Taking children into care is a last resort, and even then, more than half of the children will be looked after or fostered for short periods before returning to their birth family.

Whatever the circumstances, any parent who has lost parental responsibility for their child, whether contact is kept open or not, has experienced a tremendous loss. It is not uncommon for mothers to go on and have another child to replace the one that was lost, only to face the prospect that this child could also be taken into care. For the women who live with this loss, it is a grief as sharp as that caused by the death of a loved one, but without finality and resolution.

Ritual for Containing Difficult Feelings

If your child is taken away, whether or not you contested the decision, you are likely to have overwhelming and sometimes conflicting feelings which all need to be given space for expression. The beauty of this ritual, which is inspired by an idea of Joanna Macy's,[34] is that each feeling gets its turn.

Choose four objects to represent anger, sadness, love and hope. For example, you might choose a sturdy stick to represent anger, a bowl of water for sadness, a heart-shaped cushion for love and a lighted candle for hope.

Set aside a period of time, and if possible, ask someone to be a witness.

Make a circle using scarves laid end to end, a length of rope, or pebbles placed at intervals. Enter the circle and spend time with

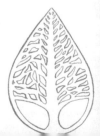

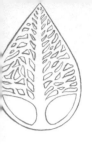

each object expressing the feelings and thoughts associated with that object's emotion. For example, with the stick, your sentences would begin: "I am angry / enraged / bitter / jealous / livid". With the water your sentences would begin: "I am sad / pained / grieved / miserable / depressed". With the heart-shaped cushion you would express your love and your longings. With the candle you would articulate the best you could imagine for yourself, your child and the whole situation. You can work in any order, and move between the objects freely. You may find that you spend nearly all the time with one object, but the others are there nevertheless, holding a space for the other emotions.

When the time allowed is over, your witness will let you know, and feed back to you anything they noticed. Then undo the circle and return your room to its normal layout. You could keep the objects to use again at regular intervals or as the need arises.

The rituals of separation are similar to those needed after a death. One birth mother kept her daughter's entire bedroom as a shrine after their parting. For a period of time this might be appropriate but after a while it may be a sign of an unrealistic hope that the child will return. Perhaps, in time, it may be possible to sift through the child's belongings for a few treasured possessions and keep these in a special box, before clearing the room. What is to be aimed at in the long term is a subtle interplay of remembering and forgetting. The child's birthdays are likely to be times of remembering. If you have a box of objects belonging to your child this could be a time to open it and contemplate with the objects inside. If you have contact with your child you could write a letter. If not, you could say the following blessing, imagining your words travelling through the world and reaching the ear of your child. Perhaps you could buy birthday cake candles and light the right number. The candles can also be pressed into earth or sand, instead of a birthday cake.

(Light 8 birthday cake candles)

Dear Katy,

You are now 8 years old, and I remember you.

I remember you when you were first born, and I remember you now on your birthday.

I wonder how your year has been. I wonder what you have learnt and who has been with you. I am still so sad not to be able to be with you. I wish I could have brought you up and looked after you but it was not possible (say the reasons . . .). Instead, I did the best I could do for you. I gave you into the hands of those who could care well for you.

In this your 8th year, I send you my love.

May you thrive. May you be happy. May you know that you are deeply loved.

Visualisation: imagine the child surrounded by the love of his or her foster / adoptive family, and also surrounded by your love.

Go well, and may my love protect you.
Go well, and may my love protect you.
Go well, and may my love protect you.

(Blow the candles out)

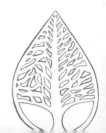

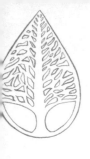

The anniversaries of the Court Orders are likely to be difficult times too. Perhaps on this day you could make a commitment to nurture yourself and send love to the person you were as you went through the separation. You could even write yourself a sealed letter, to be opened on the same day next year. This is a good way to build a supportive relationship with yourself, especially useful if you have been through a traumatic time.

These rituals can be done any time the need is felt to 'do something'. Current research suggests that people are often hit by a reaction to a trauma around eight years after the event. There could be another life event, such as becoming pregnant, or suffering another loss, which triggers the unresolved feelings. There is no shame in attending to your own need to mourn, however long it goes on. When you no longer need to hold these rituals of remembrance, they will naturally fall away.

For Adoptive Parents

Preparation for adopting

When a couple comes to adopt, they often have a history of infertility and disappointment that needs to be worked through to make a space in their lives for an adoptive child. Sue Cowling, Deputy Director and Training Manager at the Post Adoption Centre, counsels couples who are planning to adopt, using ritual to help them come to terms with past losses in preparation for adoption.

"I take a history of their losses, including miscarriages, abortions, bereavements, all the grief they are carrying. I see the couple together and individually, and we spend time going through the various stages of grief.

Then I ask the couple to imagine the ideal child that would have been born to them. I ask whether they hoped to have a boy or a girl, what the child looked like, what its talents might have been, what they would have done together. I ask them to give this mythical child a name. They write down the answers and then they talk about it together. People are often surprised at how much of a picture they have been carrying. Then I ask them to perform some kind of ritual to let go of this ideal child. Some people write poems, some make a memory box containing things belonging to a child that died. Many couples plant something as a memorial. One artist made a sculpture, and one couple cast an object into the sea.

It is important to have some kind of a ritual to say goodbye to this child for two reasons. Firstly, once you have had a 'funeral' you have permission to return to start living again. Secondly, if you let go of this ideal child, you are freer to bond with a different child who cannot replace your own child, but who adds to the family.

Often this work is done retrospectively; although addressing the issue before adoption is an ideal, it is never too late. Before going on to adopt, I lost two babies, who were born prematurely. My son was born at 28 weeks and died after three days. I did nothing ritually at the time to mark the death. It wasn't until my husband died, 20 years later to the day, that I did something. In our local cemetery we planted a rhododendron, which was significant because they grew all around the cottage where we loved to go on holiday in Somerset, and they were just coming into flower at that time of year. We had a plaque put up and I decided to add my son's name to the plaque. By

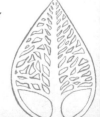

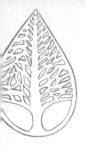

this time I had adopted children, and I talked to them about him.

My daughter was stillborn at 23 weeks, and the hospital staff recommended that I didn't look at her. Because I hadn't seen her, it never occurred to me to say that I had lost a daughter. I just blanked it. It wasn't until 30 years later, when I had done a lot of counselling training, that I decided to mark her death. I got a birth certificate from the Stillbirth and Neonatal Death Society. I had used her name for my first adopted daughter, but someone suggested I call her something different, which I did. On the anniversary of her birth and death, 30 years later, I lit a candle and put some flowers out. It was such a lovely feeling when I finally claimed her."

Adoption Day

The day when an adoption is made legal in a judge's chambers brings certainty and permanence after what is often a protracted process. The adoptive parents, and other family members, the child to be adopted, and the Social Worker will all be there as parental responsibility is signed over to the adoptive parents. This can also happen when a stepmother or father formally adopts a child from a former marriage. In some ways the court event is like a marriage, where a family is legally constructed. It is a profound moment, and yet it is a dry judicial process, in an atmosphere that may be quite tense, and in a setting where other difficult court cases may be being heard next door. The whole experience can be quite intimidating for a child. In addition, it is not possible to know in advance whether the Adoption Order will be passed, since the adoption may be contested, or there may be delays. In spite of these difficulties, many families take steps to make this occasion special and memorable.

Sally: "Beth was 10 when she was placed with us, and had lived with us for quite a while before the Adoption Order was passed. On the day, we dressed up for the occasion. After the courtroom we had photographs taken of all of us as a family. I bought a new photo frame and put her photo in the space next to the one of my other daughter. It was a symbol of her joining the family."

Other families had informal parties with the things that all children enjoy, such as going out for a meal, having cake and gifts. Although not available in mainstream shops, a range of 'Congratulations on your Adoption' cards can now be bought from www.AdoptionUK.com.

Some families continue to mark this anniversary each year, so that the child is celebrated on their birthday and also on Adoption Day. For the Davis family it became a tradition to go out for a meal on 'Davis Day' each year, even after the children were grown up and had families of their own.

Additional Ceremonies

Some families choose to welcome their adopted child through another ceremony, with more opportunity for warmth and celebration than is offered by the court procedure.

Maggie and her husband Peter were members of the Church of England, and wanted to welcome their adopted daughter into the church in a formal way. They found that there was no service available, and so wrote some words of their own:

After an opening prayer in which the birth parents were remembered, the vicar posed a series of questions to the family.

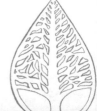

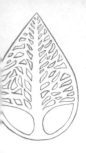

Vicar: Will you be to this child a true father and mother and brother and sister in spirit and deed?
Reply: We will.

Vicar: Will you have her in your home, and care for her in all things, as your own daughter and sister and never forsake her?
Reply: We will.

Vicar: Will you teach her by word and example the true knowledge and love of the Lord?
Reply: We will.

Then every member of the family laid a hand on the child and said,

> "We receive this child into our family with joy.
> Through God's love she comes to us,
> with God's love we will care for her,
> by God's love we will lead her
> and in God's love may we all abide forever. Amen"

The vicar held the child and welcomed her to the church in a prayer, and then closed with a blessing.

Thanksgiving for the Gift of a Child

In 1999 the Church of England introduced a service called "Thanksgiving for the Gift of a Child". This is a blessing for children, including adoptive children, and does not involve baptism. Parents affirm that they receive their child "as a gift from God" and that they seek His blessing. The minister then says:

"As Jesus took children in his arms and blessed them

so now we ask God's blessing on N.
Heavenly Father, we praise you for his/her birth;
Surround him/her with your blessing
That he/she may know your love
And know your goodness all his/her days and be protected from evil."

Family Joining Ceremonies

A non-religious alternative would be to create a "Family Joining Ceremony" of your own, which could happen at home, with just the close family present, or be part of a wider welcoming party. If it is not appropriate to include the birth parents in the adoption, they and other significant carers could still be remembered in a symbolic way, for example by lighting a candle in their honour. Whilst this may be challenging for the adoptive family to do, it could be very helpful for the child who is trying to make sense of a broken history.

Here are some suggestions for text that might be used. I have imagined in this case that the child to be adopted is old enough to take an active role, and that there is another child already in the family. Ideally, the children should take part in devising the script. The text could be read, or repeated after someone else, if the child has difficulty reading.

I have included a change of name in this ceremony. Some adopted children may be thrilled to take on their new family name, but others may have more ambivalent feelings, so it may not be appropriate to include this. A naming ceremony could always be held at a later time. Whenever a name is changed, teachers and other people should be instructed to use the new name from that day

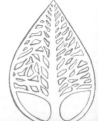

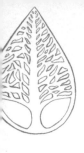

on, to reinforce the shift. Some families, as in this example, keep the child's birth parent's name as a middle name, adding their own family name at the end. Again, the child may have strong views about this.

In preparation for the ceremony, the family could decorate the room. You could ask each member of the family to bring a precious object (anything from a necklace to a teddy bear) be placed on a central table. This is a visual way of making everyone feel included. Making old-fashioned lick-and-stick paper chains provides a symbol of integration into the family, especially if each family member takes a different coloured strip.[35]

To make the event more special, children might enjoy weaving simple crowns for everyone out of thin willow or hazel branches, or out of coloured and decorated card. They could also be involved in cooking special foods for afterwards.

Family Joining Ceremony

Adoptive Parent: We are gathering today for a special occasion, to welcome Tamsin to our family.
As Kahlil Gibran has written in *The Prophet,*
"Your children are not your children.
They are the sons and the daughters of life's longing for itself"
So Tamsin, daughter of life's longing for itself, today is a special day.
Today we welcome you to the Smith family.

Tamsin: This is a special day for me too.
From today I will be a member of the Smith family.

Adoptive Parent: We acknowledge that your journey to this point has not been an easy one. We are sorry that your young life has had so much loss and sadness in it. But we also know that you have been loved and been taken care of by many people. We have a candle (or more than one) here to represent those who have loved you in the past. Would you like to light the candle(s), to remember them?

Tamsin is helped to light the candle(s)

We give thanks to everyone who has loved you and looked after you in the past. May all those who love you be blessed and held in the light.

Adoptive Parents: Now we are going to welcome you to our family. We wrap this ribbon around our wrists to show that we are joining together.

Ribbon is wrapped around the wrists of Tamsin and her adoptive mother.

Adoptive Mother: Tamsin, we welcome you, with all of your gifts and all of your history.
From today, I am your Mother.
My home is your home.
I promise to love you and care for you throughout your life.
Even if you are sad or angry, I promise to love you and care for you.
I promise to speak the truth to you,
To share with you what I love about life,
To teach you and to learn from you.

Tamsin: I promise to receive your love and care, and accept you as my mother.

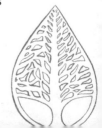

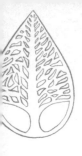

The ribbon is undone and placed on the table, and a different coloured ribbon is wrapped around the wrist of Tamsin and her adoptive father.

Adoptive Father: Tamsin, we welcome you, with all of your gifts and all of your history.
From today, I am your Father.
My home is your home.
I promise to love you and care for you throughout your life.
Even if you are sad or angry, I promise to love you and care for you.
I promise to speak the truth to you,
To share with you what I love about life,
To teach you and to learn from you.

Tamsin: I promise to receive your love and care, and accept you as my father.

The ribbon is undone and placed on the table, and a different coloured ribbon is wrapped around the wrist of Tamsin and her adoptive sister.

Tara: Tamsin, I welcome you as my new sister.
From today my Mummy is your Mummy, my Daddy is your Daddy, my home is your home.

Tamsin: Tara, I accept you as my new sister.

The ribbon is undone and placed on the table.

Adoptive Parent: To show that we are a family, we weave these ribbons together into a plait.

The three ribbons are tied at the top, plaited and tied off at the bottom. They are placed on the central table, and may later be hung from a wall.

Tamsin, now that you are a member of the Smith family, you will have a new name. Your name used to be Tamsin Ann Hobbes, and that was a good name. Now your name is Tamsin Ann Hobbes Smith and that is a good name too.

Tamsin: I used to be called Tamsin Ann Hobbes, and that was a good name.
Now my name is Tamsin Ann Hobbes Smith, and that is a good name too.

All: Welcome Tamsin Ann Hobbes Smith!

Celebratory food should follow this ceremony. A loaf of plaited bread would be particularly appropriate. On the other hand, a familiar dish may make the adopted child feel most at home. One adoptive mother told me how a meal of macaroni cheese with a tin of tomato soup on top became a special dinner for her children, after it was served to them all on a visit to their adoptive child's last foster family.

Gifts could also be given. Personalised items (e.g. jewellery or pens and pencils) using the new name might be a good idea. Children sometimes like to make and exchange friendship bracelets.

This ceremony could be adapted to include grandparents or other family members.

Entrustment Ceremonies

In the celebrations and ceremonies we have looked at so far, little mention has been made of the child's birth parents. In America, where open adoption is much more widely practised, ceremonies

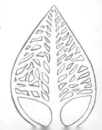

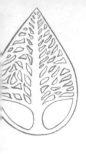

are being devised in which the birth parents are present and entrust their child to the adoptive parents. In open adoption, the birth parents stay involved with the child, but their role is significantly changed. A ritual is a good way to make this understood, not just as a concept but also as a felt reality.

At the core of an 'Entrustment Ceremony' is the moment when the birth parents physically hand over their child to the adoptive parents. Both parties then pronounce vows declaring their commitments to the child and to one another, ranging from a vow to be honest in all interactions to a vow to disclose newly discovered medical information. A social worker may record the ceremony on video so that each party, and the child, who may have been a baby at the time, has a copy to look back on.[36]

Bonding Rituals and Symbols

When welcoming a new child into the home, all kinds of everyday things can take on a symbolic dimension.

Sally: "After the Adoption Order, Beth moved in permanently. We asked what she would like in her bedroom, and she brought all her stuff from her foster home and unpacked gradually. Her toys quickly got all mixed up with Eloise's toys, and she and Eloise tried all each other's clothes on. That was clearly a part of them getting to know each other."

Other activities that give opportunities for the family to bond might be introduced deliberately. The Post Adoption Centre working with newly formed families sometimes suggest making a family shield. Using large sheets of paper and a range of pens or magazines and glue, everyone works together to decide what should be on the family shield. There might be a family motto too. Once the family shield or motto is created, it could be used on cards or even recreated in icing on a festive cake.

Planting a grafted tree in the garden, or nearby, would be a powerful way to mark an adoption. Many garden trees, from decorative maples to productive apples have a delicate sapling, bred perhaps for good fruiting or flowering, grafted onto a strong rootstock to ensure it has the best chance of thriving. As well as being a beautiful tree to be enjoyed, it may be a useful metaphor in explaining to a child about his or her adoption. (For more ideas about tree planting, see p.114.)

For the Adopted Child

However skilfully an adoption is handled, an adopted child is likely to have many confusing feelings to cope with. Just as a birth mother no longer in contact with her child needs the ceremonies of grief, an adopted child may also need to honour his feelings of loss. This is true however difficult the relationship with the birth mother has been.

One woman responded to her adopted son's two-hour temper tantrum by talking to him about how in the Jewish tradition, people sit shiva for one week when a loved one has died. During this time, other people look after their needs, and they spend time thinking and talking about the person who has died. She suggested that he could sit shiva for his lost childhood. They set aside a day for mourning, and spent it talking about the people and places he had lost, drawing pictures, playing, laughing and crying together.[37]

Difficult feelings are likely to be compounded around family days such as Christmas, Birthdays and Mother's / Father's Day. It is

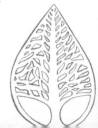

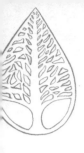

particularly tough to be full of grief and anger on a day that is supposed to be joyous, and grief can quickly become overlaid with guilt, anger and a feeling of isolation. Yet if a space is made for remembering the past and allowing grief on these occasions, it is much more likely that the child will be able to enter more fully into the festivities. The child might like to light a candle, pick a bunch of flowers or draw a picture / make a card in honour of their birth parents.

Adopting some of the child's former family or cultural traditions around these special days could also be an enriching experience for everyone. This is particularly key if the adoption is transracial.

Finally, given that adopted children have experienced so much disruption, they may well feel anxious at times of normal transition, such as moving house. Taking time to walk around the house and remember some of the things that happened there, saying goodbye and thank you to the house, blessing the next house and talking about what positive new things await there would be a helpful ritual. Something similar might be devised to help a child who was anxious about moving to a new class or school.

Mother's Day Service

A recent contribution to the pastoral care available to those affected by adoption has come in the form of an annual multi-faith Mothering Day Service of Thanksgiving, Reconciliation and Hope, organised by various different adoption agencies in turn. The service consists of hymns, prayers and addresses for all of those affected by adoption, and includes an Islamic and a Hindu contribution. At one point in the service, the whole congregation joins in an Act of

Reconciliation. Each person is given a length of ribbon and invited to write on it the name of someone touched by adoption, whom they wish to remember. The ribbons are tied to one another, and joined to those from previous years.[38]

* * *

It was after I gave a talk about ceremonies that a member of the audience said to me, "I hope you are going to write a chapter about adoption." My heart sank slightly. I knew she was right, that there should be a chapter, but I had no personal experience of this subject and had no idea where to begin. I needn't have worried. The length of this chapter and the wealth of ideas inside it are a tribute to the compassion and wisdom of the individuals and professionals working in this area, who were kind enough to talk to me. In fact, adoption proves a rich seam to mine when searching for new ceremonies. Perhaps this is because people who are willing to create new families are the sort of people who are open to creative ideas around new family rituals. Perhaps it is because children are at the centre of adoption, and they respond so well to rituals, and to inventing them. Either way, I hope that the suggestions I have made may add something to the resources available for people on all sides of the adoption triangle.

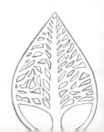

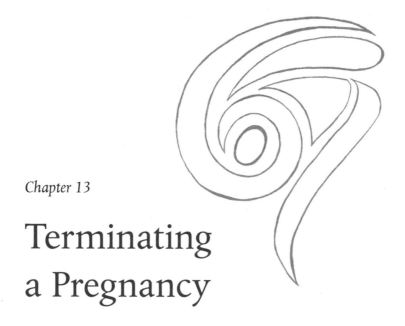

Chapter 13

Terminating
a Pregnancy

However straightforward the modern procedure for terminating a pregnancy, the decision to refuse a life is still
an awesome responsibility. The availability, speed and
comparative ease of the medical procedure belies the reality of what
is taking place. In some cases, a woman literally goes to sleep, and
when she wakes up, everything has changed. Although this degree
of distance and forgetfulness has tended to be seen in our society
as a blessing, many people, men as well as women, find that ten,
twenty, even forty years after an unmourned abortion, there is still
grief and regret, often a sense of guilt and a lack of resolution.

Creating a ritual around the experience of abortion counters this anaesthesia. The stories in this chapter are of people who wanted to remain conscious of what they were doing, and speak not about cells and tissue, but about the sons and daughters they closed the door to. Their rituals were both a way to give appropriate time and respect to their own feelings about the abortion, and also to do right by the being who was seeking incarnation. In some cases people seemed also to learn important life-lessons through the process.

Before the Termination

Some terminations are performed at a late stage, due to medical circumstances, and in these cases a strong bond may well have formed with the child already. Even when it is clear from the first that a pregnancy is not going to be welcomed, women sometimes feel a connection to the forming embryo, and begin communicating with it, perhaps through unspoken words. Sometimes the father has laid a hand on the belly and acknowledged its presence too. If some communication has already been going on, it might seem natural to continue to speak to the child, as Patricia did.

Patricia: "Before the termination I was talking to the child, preparing it. I was explaining what was going to happen, calming it down, saying I'm sorry; it's not going to be nice. I felt it was really important that I wasn't just throwing it away as rubbish."

Some midwives report that just talking to the intelligence of the forming embryo and explaining that it's not a good time and place to be, has resulted in a spontaneous miscarriage. At the very least, it gives the being some chance to prepare itself for the shock about to come.

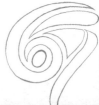

After the Termination

If you know from the outset that you wish to perform a ritual after the termination, you can ask for the remains of the foetus or request a burial.

This is what Angus and Lydia did. Remarkably, even though their relationship was ending at the time of the termination, they agreed to go through this whole process together. To honour both of their journeys, I give both their stories.

Angus: "I'd had a termination before, with another partner. We didn't do anything ritually for it, and I'm still haunted by that ghost. I feel you have to do something to mark the occasion; otherwise you're not going to have learnt from the experience. It was about respecting the potentialities that were terminated. Giving some kind of a funeral to the aborted tissue felt more respectful than throwing it in a hospital bin. Also, for me, it was about recognising that I was a 'lust child' – I should have been aborted, but I wasn't.

I wanted to do the ritual in a place where we could make a fire, and which had a view from a high place. If I were a ghost I'd want that. I carried everything that I needed – food, water, warm clothing, saw, bedding, my twenty-year-old yew staff, and the foetus in its little pot in my rucksack – and I walked from my home to the woods. The journey was the most important bit. It was timeless: the rhythm of the walking, the stick on the ground, the sweat of going uphill. After twenty minutes the daily stuff in your head recedes and you get to what is really important. I used that journey as the process for making peace, for taking responsibility for my child. Part of that was remembering how wonderful it is to be alive. Having made the choice not to give life to this child, I have to celebrate my own life, and make a commitment to living my life the best I can.

I walked around the woods for hours, finding a good spot to be. Then I gathered wood, made a fire, and when it was hot enough we burnt the foetus. I made my peace with the child, basically saying I'm sorry, and asking for peace. I took a few drops of the blood and let my staff absorb them. It was a way of asking that some of the energy of this life not lived might come into my life in a positive way. That the child's spirit might be an ally, and the experience integrated into my life.

And I made my peace with Lydia. Whatever happens, we'll have this connection – having dealt with this together. That's more than most couples have when they split up. I felt calm and peaceful afterwards in a way that surprised me. I felt I had done totally the right things; it was beyond my expectations.

Lydia: "When a friend of mine had an abortion she buried the embryo near a tree, and I had supported her to do that. I had thought of burying mine too, so I asked at my first appointment at the clinic if I could take the remains away. They made a couple of phone calls to check this was OK, and agreed. I thought I would get all the blood, but because I just asked for the 'pregnancy tissue' they just gave me the little clot and part of the placenta, in a tiny pot like a film canister, wrapped around with tape.

It was Angus who suggested cremating it rather than burying it. I didn't mind how it happened. I just wanted to mark the event. I wanted to look at it, touch it, not try to pretend that it wasn't anything it wasn't. I wanted to take full responsibility, and a cremation or burial ceremony was a way to acknowledge the life that had been.

We went to a nearby woodland and Angus chose a place, cut firewood and made a fire. We were there as the sun went down and the full moon came up. We opened the pot and looked at the embryo, and touched it, and then we put it on the fire. Seeing it sitting on a stick and sizzling, the way blood and guts do, was much harder than I thought it would be.

There were no words. My thoughts were about sending the spirit back to the spirit world, and making an apology – sorry that I wasn't able to welcome you, to take care of you, to give birth to you.

We sat for a long time just staring at the fire. The nice thing about the fire was that it gave us a period of time. If you make a burial it's over very quickly and there's nothing further to do. With a fire, you have to stay until it burns out so there is time. We talked about the end of our relationship, and how for a few days we had been a family. It was hard, but really good to do. It felt complete."

A Tibetan Buddhist Ceremony

Patricia and Jamil were travelling in Australia when they had an unplanned pregnancy leading to a termination. Shortly afterwards they began living and working in a Tibetan Buddhist Centre and whilst there, it was suggested they might like to take part in a Buddhist ceremony to address the abortion. In Buddhist terms abortion is seen as taking a life, and taking a life is seen as something that is done in ignorance. Thus their ritual centres on the expression of regret and a resolve never to do it again. The ceremony was developed by the nuns in response to a request from a therapist who had found that many of her clients were still in distress about abortions from their pasts. It can be performed at any stage after an abortion.

The ceremony begins with a visualisation of Green Tara, a manifestation of the Buddha's omniscience, love and compassion, who is called on to surround the couple and the baby with light. Prayers for the happiness of the people present and all sentient beings are said. Then the couple are asked to feel regret for any negative actions committed and asked to resolve never to do them again. They make a vow to save lives wherever possible, and to follow a spiritual path. They pray for the well-being of the 'consciousness that was their baby' asking that the baby receive whatever it needs for complete happiness. The last part of the ceremony is a visualisation of purifying light reaching the baby, the couple and all sentient beings, liberating them all from suffering, and finally becoming one with Tara.

Patricia: "We went to the nun's room, where she had a shrine to Green Tara, to help with visualisation. Mostly, the nun chanted the mantras, quite fast and rhythmically, turning to us to ask the questions. One of the hardest things was to resolve that you're never going to do it again.

Part of the ceremony is a resolution to save lives, whenever possible. The nun gave an example of a couple that had paid a fishing boat not to go out for the day. When we were in Thailand we bought frogs and toads from the market and set them free. More recently, I adopted a white cat because otherwise it would have died. I really try not to kill things now. There is a joy that comes, every time I save a life. It's very strong.

Another wonderful part of the ceremony is to wish the child well. We visualised sending golden light to the baby.

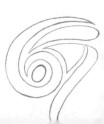

The ceremony inspired me. It healed the guilt and regret and replaced them with feelings of joy, well-being, love for myself and others, and a wish to save lives."

Jamil: "I felt touched by the ritual, but also like a passenger at times. I would have liked to be involved from a more proactive position. I think I felt a clash between my previous belief in choice on the question of abortion and the Buddhist belief of not taking any life whatever. I still believe that abortion is better sometimes than wrecking a bunch of lives. I don't know if I could do it again though. Since then I have lived with the idea that my next pregnancy would lead to a birth and this has led me closer to the idea of being a father.

I think it was helpful at the time. The only thing framing the experience before that was the waiting room of a god-awful anonymous clinic in the industrial outskirts of a grim town. Very dehumanising. So, I would say to anyone in the position we were in: yes, do it, or do something."

Mizuko Koyo – a Japanese Ritual

In Japan, since the 1970s, rituals following an abortion have become commonplace. The tradition is to buy a particular statue, called a 'mizuko' and place it in a shrine, together with a full written apology to the aborted foetus. Dolls, bibs, teddy bears and other children's items are often left with the mizuko. Prayers are made and money offered to the temple. Mizuko means "child of the waters", and the aborted foetuses are visualised as children living on a riverbank in the other world. The ritual dedicates the child to a deity, usually Jizo, who is the compassionate Bodhisattva, known as the guardian of children in the other world.

Yvonne Rand,[39] a Zen Buddhist priest and meditation teacher, who lives in the San Francisco Bay area, spent time in Japan studying the Jizo practises and has developed a ceremony for groups of people who have experienced the death (by any means) of foetuses or babies.

"The ceremony is as follows: we sit in silence, sewing a bib or hat for one of the compassion figures on the altar. The figures are from different cultures: Jizo, Mary with Jesus, "Spirit entering and leaving" from the Eskimo people, or a mother and child. Our commitment is to listen to those who wish to talk without attempting to give advice or comfort. The principle of 'no crosstalk' offers safety from uninvited comforting and solicitude, and many find it to be the most healing of possible attentions.

After this, we walk to the garden, form a circle, and go through a simple ceremony of acknowledging a particular life and death. One by one, each person says whatever is in his or her heart while offering incense, placing the sewn garments on one of the altar figures and bowing. We then chant the Heart Sutra, give the unborn beings Dharma names and say goodbye to them.

Prayer sticks are made and inscribed with prayers for forgiveness and for the wellbeing of those who have died. No names are signed. The prayers are hung from the bushes and trees in the meditation garden, thus committing our messages to the wind and the rains. Afterwards we have a cup of tea, walk in the garden, and go home with a quieter heart."

Ritual after Terminating a Pregnancy

If you have kept the pregnancy tissue from the termination, you could consider a tender earth burial, or cremation on a fire, as in the powerful story earlier in this chapter. For this ritual, however, I have imagined that there are no actual remains, and that a symbolic object will be used instead. Here the object is offered to the element of water. In our temperate climate, everyone lives within reach of some kind of watercourse, whether it is a drainage channel, broad river or ocean. Water connects intimately with the emotions, and is also a universal symbol of Life. The flow of water can liberate the flow of healing tears in ourselves; its passionate turbulence may mirror our own feelings. The emotions brought up by a pregnancy termination are likely to be strong, and a sense of blame, guilt and shame likely to be amongst them. These need to be honoured, within the embrace of compassion and forgiveness.

First, find some natural materials with which to make an object representing your potential child. You could use unbaked clay, which would dissolve quite quickly in the water, or sticks and straw, with a little wool to tie them together, which would break down more slowly. While you are making, there is an opportunity to connect with your feelings around the time of the brief pregnancy and termination, and to communicate with your image of the soul of the child. It doesn't matter if this is, for you, a real spiritual entity, or just the potentiality of a child that might have come into life.

When your figure is finished, you might want to spend some time with it before you commit it to the water, or it might feel right to do so straight away. When you are ready, go to a place near the water, and spend a little time, really watching the flow. Let it speak to you of the impermanence of the world we take for granted, and the cleansing flow of emotions and states of mind, which pass through and pass through.

Give your symbolic object to the water, in silence or with your own words of regret and love. It would be powerful to read a poem, such as Gwendolyn Brooks' *The Mother*.[40] At a time like this, poetry turns an individual sorrow into a shared piece of humanity, and makes one feel less lonely.

Pray that as your symbolic object dissolves in the water your child may be set free from this brief incarnation, and that your own difficult feelings will pass through, leaving you with forgiveness and love alone.

Marking the Due Date and Anniversaries

Some people keep with them a sense of the course of the pregnancy, and have a strange feeling around the date when the aborted baby would have been born. If a ritual was undertaken at the time of termination, it could be helpful to mark the due date with a quiet walk back to the same spot, perhaps bringing some flowers. Anniversaries of the termination may also be difficult days. An act of remembrance may be needed, such lighting a candle, bringing in flowers, meditating on compassion or giving yourself an opportunity to speak to the soul of the child again.

Grandparents

It is not often recognised that when a pregnancy is terminated, would-be grandparents may also suffer a loss.

Maggie: "We lit a candle on the anniversary of my daughter's

abortion. It was an experience that was only redeemed by being present at the birth of her next child."

* * *

The debate about the rights and wrongs of abortion, and the moment at which an embryo becomes a person with rights of their own, is set to go on and on. In the midst of that, where people are struggling with their own very difficult decisions, or mistakes, a compassionate approach to all the parties involved can only be helpful.

I say all the parties, because this chapter has accorded some status to the foetus. It has been talked about variously as a potentiality, a soul and a child. The mystery of consciousness is such that we cannot with certainty say when a collection of cells has its own life, but we should not let that hold us back from making these rituals. Maybe there is a soul you are communicating with, or maybe it's just an idea in your own mind. Either way, this work is powerful and healing, and the beauty of it is that going ahead as if the child could hear your words is enough.

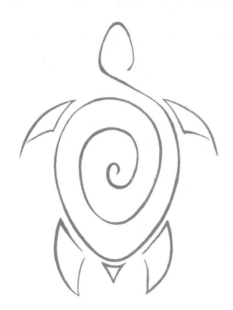

Chapter 14

Not Having Children

Although most of this book is about people consciously choosing to have children, this chapter covers the counterpart – consciously creating a life without children. People arrive at this scenario willingly or unwillingly, by very different means. Some have tried to have children and not been able, or have had to undergo a hysterectomy or sterilisation for medical reasons. Others made a positive choice not to have a family, wishing to prioritise other aspects of their life. Some women arrive at the menopause and simply have not found the right partner at the right time. Rituals for women at the menopause constitute a whole other life passage, which deserves lengthier treatment than is possible here. This chapter looks specifically at rituals for setting down the idea of having a family.

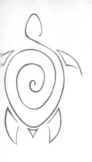

It might seem that those who have chosen childlessness would face very different issues to those who have been denied children. Certainly, there are people for whom the decision not to have children is so self-evident that any kind of ritual would be irrelevant. But people who have thought hard about it, and fought their biology not to reproduce, in the end face a similar set of circumstances. There are losses as well as gains. And there is the challenge of generating a positive image of oneself in the role of adult, without being a parent.

Choosing not to have Children

The choice not to have children is an issue for both men and women, but is probably a more challenging decision for a woman, because the capacity to bear children is so fundamental to a woman's body and psyche. In the past not having children was hardly an option for a woman, unless she remained celibate or was infertile. These days, due to more reliable birth control, having children is far more a matter of choice. People are marrying later, or not at all, and may want to prioritise their career or creativity. Some make a political decision, bearing in mind the impact of population growth on the world's resources. Some who have lived through traumatic childhoods have no wish to pass on this experience.

I talked to Chelly, a radical visual artist in her 50s, who told me her story. The ritual ideas that follow were devised through conversation between us.

Chelly: "I made the decision when I was about 35 that I wouldn't have children. I just knew that I had a different path; something else was being moved through me and I didn't want to dissipate my energy for my work. I've only got one life, one body, and I just felt I didn't have time to have children. When my mother died, I revisited the decision not to continue the lineage. At that time I had to feel it and mourn it again, but I didn't change my mind.

Although the decision wasn't agonising, I knew that if I were to hold to it I would need to gather witnesses around me who would trust my decision, and support me to feel the losses and mourn them. There are all kinds of losses. The biology has to be honoured: in a way, I still grieve every month when my period comes. There is the loss of having a relationship with a child of your own. There is the loss of not being part of a family. Also, you lose an opportunity to explore your own childhood again through the experiences of your children. I needed my decision to be affirmed as a wise choice for me. I didn't want to discuss it, or be talked out of it. I wanted it to be celebrated."

What Chelly makes clear is that even when the decision is made voluntarily, an element of grief for the path not taken may still be present. She also expresses the need to be celebrated in her choice to contribute to society in ways other than bringing up children. A woman who becomes pregnant takes on a new role and experiences a major shift in her self-image, and in how she is viewed by society. A woman who doesn't become a mother has more of a challenge to assert her worth. A man too will have to counter the suggestion that not being a father makes him a 'puer aeternis'. For this reason, the following ritual includes symbols of power for men and women to work with, in order that their decision not to have children may not feel like a loss of potency, but rather a way of channelling creative energy in a different direction.

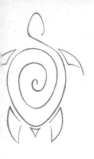

Ritual for a Life without Children

This ritual involves making two dolls, one to symbolise the losses and one the gains of not having children. With each doll, you need a little time for the making, so that you can focus your thoughts and feelings on what you are doing. The ritual also involves a symbolic burial. You will need to dig a small hole in the ground, so give some thought to where you would like this to be.

You can create each doll from straw, or clay, or anything that appeals to you, and dress it however you wish, but bear in mind that the first doll will be returned to the elements, so the materials used need to be biodegradable.

Although for clarity I have set out this ritual in two stages, you may find that working on the two dolls happens simultaneously, as the processes of grieving and celebrating intertwine.

A doll for the children not conceived

With this doll, you are making a representational image of the child or children you might have given birth to. It does not have to be a 'good' representation; its purpose is only to express your feelings. It might simply be a stick that you find and decorate. As you do this, you may find you want to give the symbolic child a name. There might be more than one doll, if you had imagined more than one child. If you have experienced miscarriages or pregnancy terminations in the past, include a doll for each of these lost children.

When the doll is ready, and when you are ready to say goodbye to it, create a quiet space to spend time with it. At this point, invite a trusted friend to be alongside you, if possible. Tell the story of how you made the doll the way it is and what you notice now you see it.

If you like, speak to the doll, saying anything that occurs to you in the moment.

Take the doll to the place where you are going to make the burial. Take your time to dig a hole and line it with whatever natural materials present themselves, such as leaves, feathers and moss. Carefully lay the doll inside and cover the grave with earth. You can scatter flowers on top, and spend as long there as you need. When you are ready, make the journey home.

Just as after a normal funeral, good nourishment and warm company will be needed to refill the places that have given up their grief. See if you can arrange for someone else to prepare a hot bowl of soup and a good hug for you on your return.

A doll for new opportunities

Now you are ready to begin making your second doll, articulating the qualities you hope to draw towards yourself in your childfree future. For example: a clear focus for the things you care passionately about; good health and abundant energy; successful creative projects; positive relationships with children and young people. Make, dress and adorn this doll to represent these qualities. When it is finished, keep this doll in a place of honour where it will inspire you regularly.

Symbols of Power for Men and Women

By conceiving a child, new mothers and fathers take on the mantle of parenting, linking them in a chain that stretches for generations behind them, and, at least one generation before them. Instead of

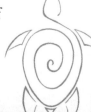

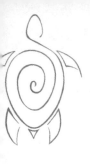

this, you might like to meditate on the spiritual forbears and mentors that have inspired you to get to where you are today. Visualise these people standing behind you, smiling on you and offering you support. Now meditate on the ways in which your presence in the world influences the next generation. See all the individuals whom you teach, mentor or influence, standing in front of you and receiving your support, and perceive the goodwill from them moving on into the next generation.

To turn this image into a visible form, you could give yourself a gift of a ceremonial cloth or scarf to express your sacred inheritance in the world, your sovereign judgement, and your good guardianship. This is an invitation to find, make or buy yourself such a garment, just for you, as a treat.

If you are a woman who has decided not to offer her womb to be a vessel within which a new human life will form, you might consider in what other ways you would still want to be receptive and fertile. As a meditation on receptivity, you could find, make or buy for yourself a beautiful vessel – a shell, vase, jug, cup, bowl or cooking pot – that represents your openness to life.

If you are a man who has decided not to father children, you might consider the ways in which you might use your strength and abilities to protect the vulnerable and champion truth. A staff – again found, made or bought – could be a useful focus for this awareness.

In an ideal world, you might find a respected friend to present you with these gifts, perhaps at a birthday party. Whenever you use these sacred objects, they will serve to remind you of your resolve to be powerful and generous. When not in use, they could be placed together with your doll for new opportunities to form a little shrine in your house as a place to go with your prayers for guidance and direction.

* * *

Given that deciding not to have children, or coming to terms with not having them, is something that one lives with and revisits over a period of many years, there is no right time-scale or order in which to approach these activities. Different ideas could be used at different times, whenever a need is felt. Finally, as with all ritual work, the dolls and other objects are a reminder to the unconscious which direction you want to move in, they are not a short-cut to being there.

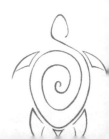

Conclusion

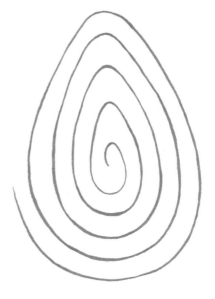

A common theme in all of the ceremonies and meditations this book has described or proposed, is that they are made by the people, not written down in a venerated book. This is interesting. As people drift away from the rituals handed down to them, a creative space is opened up. An opportunity presents itself to look within, to search and experiment and devise new forms with which to express our deepest needs and longings. There are people confident and articulate enough to take this on, and we do not, at the moment, risk being imprisoned for heresy or burnt at the stake for witchcraft if we do. Never before have we had so much freedom to make our own ceremony. And, given that a ceremony is a small slice of time within which we can fashion an ideal world, never before have we had so much power to revision reality.

Making new ceremonies is part and parcel of a wider movement by people who are seeking alternatives to unsustainable and dehumanising practises in all areas of life, not just by lobbying governments for change but also by doing things themselves. Whether we are talking about building houses, growing food, or bringing up children, there is a hearty and growing number of people who believe that the systems in place have been built on faulty foundations and there is an urgent need to do things differently. It is no co-incidence that there is a resurgence of interest in ceremony amongst the same kind of people who work to promote sustainability in agriculture or cooperative work practises. All of these activities are profoundly counter-cultural. Even the choice to make a baby greetings card rather than buying one from a shop is a choice against bland consumerism and in favour of uniqueness and diversity. Ours is less an age of rebellion than a time for radical creativity on all fronts. Of course, only some of these 'alternatives' are really new. There is just as much that is being remembered and borrowed from pre-modern systems, when humans, by necessity, lived in a closer, more tangible relationship to their environment. This is as true of organic agriculture as it is of 'new' ceremony that often borrows ideas from Native American or Celtic pre-Christian origins.

In our fragmented and multiple society, we will increasingly need to find new ways of coming together in common purpose. Even within one family there may be a collision of backgrounds, cultures and beliefs, and I think this is a good thing. It will force us to reach for a new language of symbols and words that express what is universal as well as what we each hold dear. Self-penned ceremony is more flexible than traditional ritual, unencumbered by power structures that maintain the status quo. This makes it well

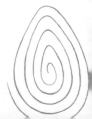

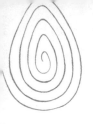

suited to bringing together people from many faiths or none, in conventional or unconventional families, and building community around an appreciation of common humanity. What could be more human, or more important, than to sing, to share food together, to celebrate when we are blessed and to console one another when we experience loss?

What is more, the very struggle to include everybody, and the work that goes into making a family event, is a way of weaving the cloth of community. This happens in very simple practical ways: a relative is asked to find a poem they love, another brings the cake, a friend offers skills in dressmaking and someone else takes photographs, but the whole is greater than the sum of the parts. One thing that makes community work, and that makes people happy, is when people are able to contribute their skills and time to a project in a way that is appreciated. Our society is set up in such a way that our opportunities to be creative in a direct way are very limited. Exquisite music is available on recordings, clothes made the other side of the world are cheap to buy, cakes can be picked up in a supermarket. Meanwhile, we often spend our days doing distant and ethereal things to make a living, and hardly have the energy to cook dinner when we get home. The joy of a hand-made ceremony is that our skills are actually needed. Even if it isn't practical to make all our own clothes all the time, we push the boat out for a special outfit for a bride or baby. Decorating a cake can provide a glorious opportunity for fun, even, given encouragement, by someone who professes to be 'no good at that sort of thing'. When we sing together, we feel the resonance of song in the heart, rather than leaving that pleasure only for the professionals. It's not about being the best, it's just about making something beautiful, and doing it in collaboration with other people.

Which leads me on to talking about celebrants. There are one or two organisations whose stated aim is to train celebrants – either humanist or interfaith. However, the majority of people doing this work have, like myself, found that they've grown into it. Perhaps they were involved in theatre or other arts, used to public speaking and the creative process. Perhaps they are counsellors who understand people's need for ritual. Or perhaps they were mothers who became grandmothers and found that other people began to see them as wise ones, and ask them to help out. Sometimes they are people from within a religion who are working at the frontiers of what people within their tradition deem acceptable. For example, there is a great deal of new ceremony being created by and for Jewish women, overturning centuries of discrimination. Certainly there is skill involved in putting together and holding an event gracefully, but this role need not be the province of an expert. A good celebrant will have experience to draw on and will use it facilitate the protagonists of the ceremony to articulate the things that are important to them. The celebrant's role is one of listening, hand-holding and steering, and his status as a leader is leant by the participants for the period of the ceremony alone. Many ceremonies use the shape of a circle, where everyone can see everyone else, to emphasise the equality of the people present.

Everything I've said so far applies to all new ways of marking rites of passage, including marriages and funerals, but ceremonies for parents and babies have a particular significance when it comes to dreaming up a new and better world. Our generation and the

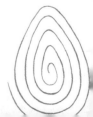

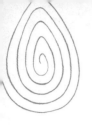

ones soon to come are going to face unprecedented challenges from climate change and human population growth, as the fact of finite planetary resources finally hits home. With full knowledge of how hard things will be, and how much each new person has an impact on the world, some people understandably choose not to have children at all. If, in spite of this knowledge, we decide we do want to make a family, we may as well do our best to bring up children who will be worth their carbon footprint. We are going to need people with bright minds, good hearts and plenty of courage to create a society in better relationship with itself and the natural world. Taking the best care possible of the parents and embryos of the next generation seems a good step towards preserving humanity. How we arrive in the world and how welcome we feel here may play a significant part in how we treat it in our lives to come. We owe it both to our children and to the world, to conceive, birth and welcome our children with as much love and prayerfulness as possible.

Fundamentally, what we are talking about here is maintaining a connection with spirit. I am not going to try and define what that means, but I think we can feel towards it. We touch spirit when we recover a sense of wonder, and when we glimpse the bigger picture of which we are a part. This time of life that I have called the 'child-bearing years' – the opening to the possibility of conception, the waiting, the bearing of children, the birthing of them, or the denial of them – is rich in spirit. That moment when new life begins is so miraculous, the experience of birth so awesome, that it can lift us into an altered state. Even the most rational of us can be filled with amazement at the thrust of life, somehow contriving to propel itself into the future, through the vessels of hapless individuals. And then there is the fact that the unruliness of our bodies' fertility merrily confounds our minds' desire to control things. Whenever we are foiled in our attempts to keep things in order, we meet with a little more reality, and can reach a more humble understanding of our place in the world.

With so many calls on our time, slowing down sufficiently to give attention to our own physical and emotional states in the ways I've suggested in this book might seem an indulgence we can ill afford. Yet if we numb ourselves to our own pain, we also cut ourselves off from our source of strength and wisdom, which leaves us flailing and making poor decisions, eating or drinking to excess, or seeking some other distraction. By contrast, when we move through our lives consciously and keep rituals, we are in good relationship with ourselves, with our families, friends and neighbours, with our ancestors and with the ones to come. Tuning in to what is really going on in our bodies, we become more aware, more composed and more compassionate. We feel as though we matter, and that helps us to remember that everyone else, everything else, matters too. Going prayerfully, we are also working with what the Native Americans call 'all our relations' and, as the Buddhists say, 'for the benefit of all beings.' If we are to have a hope of surviving as a species into the future it is imperative that we learn both how to find common purpose with our human neighbours and how to behave as part of an interconnected fabric of life. The practise of making ceremonies is earthy work, but at its most profound, this is what it can lead us to.

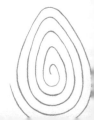

Endnotes

1 From *Snow* by Louis MacNeice 1907-1964.
2 Chant XXIX Proverbios y Cantarès, Campos de Castilla, 1917.
3 E.g. www.starchild.co.uk.
4 *Welcoming Spirit Home* Sobonfu E. Some (New World Library 1999).
5 For more information see www.arvigomassage.com.
6 *Inanna, Queen of Heaven and Earth* by Diane Wolkstein and Samuel Noah Kamer (Perennial Sept 83).
7 To see some inspirational vulva puppets see www.yoni.com.
8 From *A Kavanah for Conception* by Gershon Ellison www.ritualwell.org.
9 For more information see www.arvigomassage.com.
10 www.ritualwell.org. Reprinted from *Tikkun: A Bimonthly Jewish Critique of Politics, Culture and Society.*
11 See www.doula.org.uk for more information and a national list of qualified doulas.
12 See *The Songlines* Bruce Chatwin (Vintage 1998).
13 *Birth Traditions and Modern Pregnancy* Care Jacqueline Vincent Priya (Element 1992).
14 Quoted in *Power of Raven Wisdom of Serpent* Noragh Jones (Floris Books 1994).
15 For many more ideas of this kind, see *Birthing from Within* Pam England and Rob Horowitz (Partera Press 1998).
16 *Spiritual Midwifery* 4th edition, Ina May Gaskin (Book Publishing Company, USA 2002).
17 *Ibid.*
18 See *Cultural Awareness in Nursing and Health Care* Karen Holland and Christine Hogg (Arnold).
19 *Birth Traditions & Modern Pregnancy Care* Jacqueline Vincent Priya (Element 1992).
20 See *Childbirth Wisdom* Judith Goldsmith (Congdon & Weed Inc. 1984).
21 The 1552 Book of Common Prayer.
22 *Welcoming Spirit Home* Sobonfu Some (New World Library 1999).
23 *Ibid.*
24 *New Arrivals* published by the British Humanist Association.

25 See *Engineers of the Imagination – the Welfare State International Handbook* Baz Kershaw and Tony Coult (Methuen 1983) for how to make flags and lanterns

26 For a full account of this event see *The Dead Good Book of Naming and Baby Welcoming Ceremonies* edited by Jonathan How with Sue Gill and John Fox (Engineers of the Imagination 1999).

27 *Plants For People* by Anna Lewington (Eden Project Books 2003).

28 From *Humanistic Judaism* Winter/Spring 1999, Beth Haskala, Rochester Society for Humanistic Judaism Society for Humanistic Judaism, 28611 West Twelve Mile Road, Farmington Hills, MI 48334. Email: info@shj.org. www.shj.org.

29 See *A practical Guide to Alternative Baptism and Baby-Naming* by Kate Gordon (Constable 1998).

30 See page 85, *The Natural Death Handbook* 4th edition, edited by Stephanie Wienrich and Josefine Speyer of the Natural Death Centre (Rider 2003).

31 Some of this material was quoted in *The Natural Death Handbook* (ibid.) and is reproduced here along with new material by permission of Mary Wallace.

32 Natural Death Centre in the Hill House, Watley Lane, Twyford, Winchester SO21 1QX Tel: 0871 288 2098 www.naturaldeath.org.uk

33 Extract from a poem called *My Beautiful Butterfly* by Wanda from Swindon, published in the Natural Parents Network newsletter April 2005.

34 See *Coming Back to Life Practices to Reconnect Our Lives, Our World* Joanna Macy and Molly Young Brown (New Society Publishers 1998).

35 This is an idea suggested in *Creating Ceremonies – Innovative Ways to Meet Adoption Challenges* Cheryl Lieberman PhD and Rhea Bufferd LICSW (Zeig, Tucker & Co., Inc 1999).

36 For the full text of an Entrustment Ceremony see www.openadoptioninsight.org

37 See *Creating Ceremonies* as above.

38 For more information contact AAA-Norcap (see Resources).

39 From her article: "The Buddha's Way and Abortion: Loss, Grief and Resolution". www.buddhistinformation.com/buddha3.htm last viewed 21/7/05.

40 "The Mother'" by Gwendolyn Brooks b 1917 USA (see *Generations – Poems Betwen Fathers, Mothers, Daughters, Sons* ed. Melanie Hart and James Loader Penguin 1998 p.136)

Resources

Recommended Poems and Songs

Pregnancy

"Heartsong" by Jeni Couzyn (*Being Alive* ed. Neil Astley, Bloodaxe 2004 p 110)

"Scan at 8 weeks" by Helen Dunmore (*ibid* p 111)

"The Unborn Daughter" by R. S. Thomas (*The Nation's Favourite Poems of Childhood* ed. Alex Warwick BBC Worldwise 2000 p 33)

"To a Little Invisible Being who Is Expected Soon to Become Visible" by Anna Laetitia Barbauld (*All the Poems you Need to Say Hello* ed. Kate Clancy, Picador 2004 p 25)

Birth

"The night before the last day of January" by Kona Macphee (*All the Poems you Need to Say Hello* ed. Kate Clancy, Picador 2004 p 118)

"Tempo" by Lauris Edmond (*ibid* p 122)

"Transformation" by Jeni Couzyn (*The Nation's Favourite Poems of Celebration*, BBC Worldwide 2002 p 35)

Becoming a Father

"A Celebration" by George Macbeth (*Generations* ed. Melanie Hart and James Loader, Penguin 1998 p 16)

"The Harvest in March" by W. N. Herbert (*Being Alive* ed. Neil Astley, Bloodaxe 2004 p 119)

"To My Daughter" by Stephen Spender (*Generations* p 24)

Naming Ceremonies

"On Children" by Kahlil Gibran (*The Prophet*, Knopf 1923)

"The Mothers Song" – Inuit traditional (*Crossings* ed. Annemarie Heywood, Macmillan Education Ltd 1998 p 81)

"Woman to Child" by Judith Wright (*Poem for the Day: 366 Poems, Old and New, Worth Learning by Heart* ed. Nicholas Albery and Peter Ratcliffe, Sinclair-Stevenson 1994 p 365)

"You're" by Silvia Plath from *Collected Poems* (Faber and Faber 2003)

"On Children" Ysaye Barnwell's setting of Kahlil Gibran's words (recorded on *Sweet Honey in the Rock: Breaths* CD 1988) Also available as sheet music arranged for SSAA

"We are" by Ysaye Barnwell (recorded on *Sweet Honey in the Rock: Sacred Ground* CD, Earthbeat/Warner Brothers 1995) Also available as sheet music arranged for SATB in the Sweet Honey in the Rock Continuum Songbook

"Everything Possible", "Welcome to the World" and "It's your birthday" from the album *Why Does It Have To Be Me?* Roy Bailey with Val Bailey, Sue Harris & John Kirkpatrick (Fuse Records CFCD 396. 1989)

Miscarriage

"The Lost Baby Poem" Lucille Clifton (*Being Alive* ed. Neil Astley, Bloodaxe 2004 p 110)

Terminating a Pregnancy

"The Mother" by Gwendolyn Brooks, USA (*Generations* p136)

Stillbirth

"Child Burial" by Paula Meehan (*Generations* p 142)

Sourcebooks for Prayers, Poems and Readings

All the Poems you need to say Hello ed. Kate Clanchy (Picador 2004)

Being Alive ed Neil Astley (Bloodaxe 2004)

Generations – Poems Between Fathers, Mothers, Daughters, Sons ed. Melanie Hart and James Loader (Penguin 1998)

In the Gold of Flesh: Poems of Birth and Motherhood ed. R Palmeira (Women's Press 1990)

Life Prayers From Around the World – 365 Prayers, Blessings and Affirmations to Celebrate the Human Journey ed. Elizabeth Roberts and Elias Amidon (Harper Collins 1996)

Newborn – Poems by Kate Clanchy (Picador 2004)

Perspectives on a Grafted Tree – Thoughts for Those Touched by Adoption (Perspectives Press 1983)

Poem for the Day: 366 Poems, Old and New, Worth Learning by Heart ed. Nicholas Albery and Peter Ratcliffe (Sinclair-Stevenson 1994)

The Nation's Favourite Poems of Childhood ed. Alex Warwick (BBC Worldwide 2000)

The Prophet by Kahlil Gibran (Knopf 1923)

Recommended Books

Conception and Preconception
Welcoming Spirit Home Sobonfu E. Some (New World Library 1999)
Building Better Babies: Preconception Planning for Healthier Children Daniel Elam (Celestial Arts 1980)
How to Get Pregnant Sherman J. Silber (Warner Books 1980)
Inanna, Queen of Heaven and Earth Diane Wolkstein and Samuel Noah Kamer (Perennial Sept 83)

Pregnancy
Meditations For Your Pregnancy – Sheila Lavery and Pippa Duncan (Golden 1999)

Birth
Birthing from Within: An Extraordinary Guide to Childbirth Preparation Pam England & Rob Horowitz (Partera Press 1998)
Childbirth Wisdom Judith Goldsmith (Congdon & Weed Inc. 1984)
Power of Raven Wisdom of Serpent Noragh Jones (Floris Books 1994)
Rediscovering Birth Sheila Kitzinger (Little, Brown and Company 2000)
Spiritual Midwifery 4th edition Ina May Gaskin (Book Publishing Company 2002)
The Songlines Bruce Chatwin (Vintage 1998)

Naming Ceremonies
A practical guide to Alternative Baptism and Baby-Naming – Kate Gordon (Constable and Co 1998)
Engineers of the Imagination – the Welfare State International Handbook Baz Kershaw and Tony Coult (Methuen 1983)
From Beginning to End Robert Fulghum (Rider Books 1995)
Plants For People by Anna Lewington (Eden Project Books 2003)
The Dead Good Book of Namings and Baby Welcoming Ceremonies – ed. Jonathon How with Sue Gill and John Fox (Engineers of the Imagination (1999)
Welcoming Spirit Home Sobonfu Some (New World Library 1999)

Adoption
Creating Ceremonies. Innovative Ways to Meet Adoption Challenges by Cheryl A. Lieberman, Ph.D. and Rhea K. Bufferd, LICSW (Zieg, Tucker & Co, Phoenix, Arizona 1999)
Coming Back to Life: Practices to Reconnect Our Lives, Our World by Joanna Macy and Molly Young Brown (New Society Publishers 1998)

Organisations

AAA-NORCAP
112 Church Road, Wheatley, Oxfordshire OX33 1LU
Tel: 01865 875000 www.norcap.org.uk
Providing support for adults affected by adoption, including support with searching and being reunited with birth relatives.

Adoption UK
46 The Green, South Bar Street, Banbury OX16 9AB
Tel: 01295 752240 Helpline 0844 8487900 (10am – 4pm)
www.AdoptionUK.com
A national self-help group run by and for adoptive parents and foster carers, offering support before, during and after adoption.

Birth Crisis Network
A network of people who can be telephoned if you have experienced a traumatic birth. See www.sheilakitzinger.com/BirthCrisis.htm to find the regional contact nearest you.

British Infertility Counselling Association
111 Harley Street, London W1G 6AW
Tel: 01372 451626
www.bica.net
Professional association for infertility counsellors in the UK. Their website can help you find a counsellor locally.

Care Confidential
Clarendon House, 9-11 Church Street, Basingstoke RG21 7QG
Helpline (freephone) 0800 028 2228 www.careconfidential.com
Offers counselling, help and advice to those who find themselves facing an unplanned pregnancy or who are concerned after an abortion.

Child Death Helpline
Helpline Freephone 0800 282986 www.childdeathhelpline.org.uk
The Child Death Helpline is a helpline for anyone affected by the death of a child of any age, from prebirth to adult, under any circumstances, however recently or long ago.

Doula UK
PO Box 26678, London N14 4WB
Tel: 0871 433 3103 www.doula.org.uk
The non profit association for doulas in the UK, including lists of doulas to help you find one in your area.

The Environment Agency
Tel: 08708 506 506 to be directed to your nearest regional office
www.environment-agency.gov.uk
To be contacted if you are considering a burial on private land or for advice
on scattering ashes.

Foresight Preconception
Head Office, 178 Hawthorn Road, Bognor Regis, West Sussex PO21 2UY
(01243) 868001 www.foresight-preconception.org.uk
Offers hair analysis and comprehensive advice on optimum health for
preconception.

Insight
www.openadoptioninsight.org
American organisation offering resources and support for people engaged in
open adoption, where the adopted child maintains a relationship with their
birth family.

The Miscarriage Association
c/o Clayton Hospital, Northgate, Wakefield
West Yorkshire WF1 3JS
Helpline: 01924 200799 (Mon-Fri, 9am-4pm)
www.miscarriageassociation.org.uk

Natural Death Centre
In the Hill House, Watley Lane, Twyford, Winchester SO21 1QX
Tel: 0871 288 2098 www.naturaldeath.org.uk
Gives advice & support on family-organised, environmentally-friendly
funerals, and Natural Burial Grounds.

Natural Parents Network
18 Bishops Way, Stradbroke, Suffolk IP21 5JR
Helpline Tel: 0845 4565031 www.n-p-n.co.uk
A national self-help organisation for natural parents and relatives who have
lost children to adoption.

Post-Adoption Centre
5 Torriano Mews, Torriano Avenue, London NW5 2RZ
Tel: 020 7284 0555 Advice line: 020 7284 5879 www.postadoptioncentre.org.uk
Provides independent advice, counselling, training and support to anyone
affected by adoption.

Ritualwell
www.ritualwell.org
This website was set up by two American organisations, Kolot: The Centre for Jewish Women's and Gender Studies and Ma'yan: The Jewish Women's Project. It provides a wealth of resources for creating innovative contemporary Jewish rituals.

Stillbirth and Neonatal Death Society (SANDS)
28 Portland Place, London W1B 1LY
Tel: 020 7436 7940 Helpline 020 7436 5881 www.uk-sands.org
Supports anyone affected by the death of a baby and promotes research to reduce the loss of babies' lives.

Winston's Wish
General Enquiries 01242 515157 Helpline 0845 2030405
www.winstonswish.org.uk
Offers help for bereaved children and their families. Their shop stocks books and leaflets along with memorial candles, and custom made Memory Boxes.

The Woodland Trust
Autumn Park, Grantham, Lincolnshire NG31 6LL
Tel: 01476 581111 www.woodland-trust.org.uk
They run a scheme through which you can dedicate a tree or area of woodland. www.dedicatetrees.com

Celebrants and other Contacts

All the people in this list are known to the author or contributed in some way to this book. It is in no way a comprehensive list of people working as celebrants in the UK.

Hugh Dunford Wood is an artist based in Dorset who runs mentoring groups, retreats and vision quests. Contact: dunfordwood@talk21.com

Miche Fabre Lewin is an Oxfordshire-based artist and food ritualist who can co-create a unique food ceremony with deep tasting food, honouring soil, season and spirit. Contact: michefabrelewin@mac.com

Sue Gill works as a secular celebrant in South Cumbria and runs workshops about rites of passage. Together with John Fox she has written and published The Dead Good Book of Namings and Baby Welcoming Ceremonies and other books. See: www.deadgoodguides.com

Glennie Kindred is an artist, writer and celebrant in the Derbyshire area, with many years experience of creating ceremony with an earth-based/interfaith spirituality. Contact: glenniekindred@w3z.co.uk www.glenniekindred.co.uk

Karen Kay is an Oxford-based musician who sings at ceremonies and gatherings. Contact: 01865 250567 karen@wildruby.co.uk.

Liz Rothschild is a freelance celebrant based in Wiltshire. Her work, Markings, helps people to mark significant events or stages in their lives. Contact: 01367 240508.

Lizzie Ruffell is an Oxford-based birth educator offering holistic birth preparation as well as fertility, pre and post-natal massage. Contact: 01865 725776 lizzieflow@hotmail.com www.birthtides.co.uk

Margot Oakenby is based in Oxford and helps people create ceremonies for all occasions, with an emphasis on bringing spirit into everyday life. Contact: 07960 707607

Mary Wallace is a celebrant for the Humanist Society of Scotland and conducts non-religious ceremonies including funerals for babies and children. Contact: mary.wallace@humanism-scotland.org.uk

Meredith Wheeler is a psychotherapist specialising in fertility issues. She has run fertility support groups, workshops and fertility loss services for over 15 years. www.meredithwheeler.org meredith.wheeler@free.fr

Tess Ward is an Oxford-based hospital chaplain and celebrant whose work honours the spirituality of people of all faiths or none. She offers baby blessings, and has experience of blessings and funerals for babies who are stillborn or die soon after birth. Contact: 07910 320450 tess.ward@btinternet.com www.greenblessing.org.uk

Inspiration
for Self Reliance

SOME OTHER BOOKS
from
PERMANENT
PUBLICATIONS

ALL THESE & MUCH MORE AVAILABLE FROM
The Green Shopping Catalogue
www.green-shopping.co.uk
or any good bookshop

If you enjoyed this book you won't want to miss this magazine!

Permaculture Magazine helps you live a more natural, healthy and environmentally friendly life.

Permaculture Magazine offers tried and tested ways of creating flexible, low cost approaches to sustainable living. It can help you to:

- Make informed ethical choices
- Grow and source organic food
- Put more into your local community
- Build energy efficiency into your home
- Find courses, contacts and opportunities
- Live in harmony with people and the planet

Permaculture Magazine is published quarterly for enquiring minds and original thinkers everywhere. Each issue gives you practical, thought provoking articles written by leading experts as well as fantastic eco-friendly tips from readers!

permaculture, ecovillages, organic gardening, sustainable agriculture, agroforestry, appropriate technology, eco-building, downshifting, community development, human-scale economy... and much more!

Permaculture Magazine gives you access to a unique network of people and introduces you to pioneering projects in Britain and around the world. Subscribe today and start enriching your life without overburdening the planet!

Every issue of *Permaculture Magazine* brings you the best ideas, advice and inspiration from people who are working towards a more sustainable world.

Permanent Publications
The Sustainability Centre, East Meon, Hampshire GU32 1HR, UK
Tel: 0845 458 4150 or 01730 823 311 Fax: +44 (0)1730 823 322
Email: orders@permaculture.co.uk Web: www.permaculture.co.uk